Infection Control in the Dental Environment

Infection Control in the Dental Environment

Effective Procedures

Michael V Martin
BDS, BA, PhD, MRCPath

Senior Lecturer and
Consultant in Oral Microbiology,
University of Liverpool, Liverpool, UK

Martin Dunitz

First published in the United Kingdom in 1991 by
Martin Dunitz Ltd, 7–9 Pratt Street, London NW1 0AE

A CIP catalogue record for this book is available from the
British Library.

ISBN 1-85317-028-3

Phototypeset by Scribe Design, Gillingham, Kent

Printed in Great Britain by The University Press, Cambridge

Contents

Acknowledgments

No author ever writes a book without the support of friends. This book probably would not have been written without the support of Peter Woods and David Phillips. These two gentlemen shared a cross infection control lecture tour of the UK with me and, apart from being enjoyable, I learned a lot from them. Others helped as well: in particular Douglas Cochrane, of KaVo International, was a mine of information and help. The arduous job of deciphering my handwriting fell to Brenda Smith who did it with patience and thought: I thank her. Mary Banks, Lucy Hamilton and Alison Campbell of Martin Dunitz Ltd have been extremely helpful, good humoured and expeditious in getting this manuscript into production; it was a pleasure to work with them.

Finally, I should like to thank M. O'C without whom this book would have been finished two months earlier!

MVM

Preface

The whole subject of cross infection control has had a high impact on dentistry in the last 5 years. There is a plethora of published material, guidelines and anecdotal advice. In the course of 10 years' experience in lecturing about this subject in various parts of the world, I have encountered an enormous diversity of opinions and still, in some circles, apathy about the whole problem. This book is a synthesis of this experience and, it is to be hoped, a practical text which also provides the theoretical background for the whole dental team. Cross infection control is a matter of importance for everybody: operators, staff and patients.

Liverpool, 1990   **MVM**

Introduction

It is important to distinguish cross infection from contamination. Contamination is the transfer of exogenous micro-organisms to a patient. Exogenous (as opposed to endogenous) micro-organisms are those not normally found in a particular patient. Cross infection control is the sum total of all the measures taken to prevent subsequent infection. In dentistry, the techniques used have to be specially adapted so they can be easily applied to the wide range of different procedures undertaken.

It is important that such procedures are practical and easily understood and reproduced by a wide range of auxiliary staff. The control of cross infection must be economical and involve the minimum loss of surgery time. This requires planning and the purpose of this book is to help dental practitioners implement sensible, practical, safe procedures.

PRACTICAL POINTS
—for the ideal cross infection control procedures

- **Should be simple**
- **Easily reproduced**
- **Economical**
- **Should not involve a great deal of surgery time**
- **Should be easily understood by all staff**
- **Should not involve toxic substances**

An understanding of risk areas is crucial to the establishment of good cross infection control procedures. Dentistry is unusual in that it is undertaken in an environment in which there is saliva and blood. In addition, there are aerosols, splatter and the possibility of flying debris. The resheathing of local anaesthetic needles in dentistry is routine and can be a serious infection risk.

Blood is a well recognized vector of pathogenic micro-organisms and there are few, if any, dental procedures in which blood contamination is not a risk. Saliva adds a further dimension to this risk for, although it has some microbiocidal properties, it can contain large numbers of bacteria, viruses and fungi. There is also some evidence to show that certain viruses can be actively secreted into saliva.

In most European countries and the United States, the responsibility for cross infection control lies unequivocally with the practising dentist. Where a number of dentists work together in a group practice, clinic or hospital, the individual dentist who operates on the patient is still the responsible person. Law suits involving cross infection in the United Kingdom, most states of the USA and European countries usually name the operating dentist, with the head of the clinic or hospital as a secondary person in the allegation. The legal responsibility of a practising dentist is summed up by the UK Health and Safety at Work Act, which states 'that no person should as a result of conditions at the workplace be exposed to injury'.[1] This legal responsibility also involves auxiliary personnel. In a dental practice, hygienists, dental nurses, technicians and cleaning staff must all be protected by the dentist from infection. The legal responsibility for cross infection control thus extends well beyond the patients attending the surgery.

Legal claims involving cross infection control, or the lack of it, are now increasing rapidly. In the USA and the UK, legal precedents have been set for such cases. The author has had the dubious privilege of giving advice in legal cases in three states of the USA, in the UK, France and Spain. One clear legal precedent has emerged from all these cases and that is deviation from the individual state or country's professional guidelines[2,3] makes one liable to successful prosecution by patients. Thus the professional guidelines on cross infection control of individual countries are the minimum legally acceptable standards required.[2-4] The UK General Dental Council has withdrawn the practising certificate of one dentist who failed to practise satisfactory infection control. The practitioner in this case was accused and convicted of 'gross professional misconduct likely to be prejudicial to a patient's health'.

The most frightening aspect of legal cases involving cross infection is that usually it is not necessary to prove unequivocally that the illness was due to dental procedures. This may seem strange but often the illnesses involved have long incubation periods; proving the cause and the effect of the illness is often impossible. If a patient is able to show, on the balance of possibilities, that a serious risk of the transfer of micro-organisms may have resulted from dental treatment, then the dentist is usually culpable. Such judgments are in practice rare as settlement from malpractice insurance occurs long before a judgment is pronounced. Thus, if a patient is able to show that cross infection could have occurred, then the dentist may be guilty – a chilling prospect indeed.

It is therefore important to read the appropriate professional guidelines and apply them to daily practice. This book is aimed to help provide simple, straightforward and safe procedures within the guidelines.

Identification of the patient at risk

The routine use of the medical history has been advocated as the method of identification of patients capable of transmitting infectious disease. Such advocates are operating on fallacious grounds as often it is impossible to distinguish infectious patients from their medical history. This is due in part to the fact that many patients are unaware of their medical status and also that some conceal or are at best economical with the truth. If hepatitis B carriage is taken as an example, 50 per cent of patients have subclinical infections and are often unaware of their condition. Therefore, even though a patient offers a truthful medical history it is not helpful without further tests. Clearly in the confines of a dental practice, testing for hepatitis B surface (HBsAg) or e (HBeAg) antigens is impractical: however, this would be the only reliable method of identification of hepatitis B in these patients.

The situation with human immunodeficiency virus (HIV) is much more complex. Questions concerning sexual proclivities are difficult and often embarrassing to ask and in many cases simply offend these patients. If the information that a patient is promiscuously homosexual or bisexual is volunteered, it is not necessarily of help if the HIV antibody status is not known. Such information may help to form a provisional diagnosis of AIDS if symptoms including persistent generalized lymphadenopathy or intractable oral candidosis are present. This information is still not helpful unless there is positive confirmatory laboratory evidence. In some cases, this can be obtained from the laboratory investigating the patient. However, for medico-legal reasons, this information is becoming increasingly more difficult to obtain.

The solution to this quandary is to regard every patient as potentially infectious. This eliminates the necessity for two standards

Table 1.1 Important diseases in infection control

Disease	Cause	Route	Incubation period	Possible complications
Viral				
AIDS, ARC	Human immuno-deficiency virus	Parenteral blood	At least 10 months	AIDS, opportunistic infections
Chicken pox	Varicella virus	Saliva, droplets	9–22 days	Chicken pox, shingles
German measles	Rubella virus	Saliva, droplets	8–12 days	Infant death or malformation
Hepatitis A	Hepatitis A virus	Poor hygiene	2–6 weeks	Usually full recovery
Hepatitis B	Hepatitis B virus	Parenteral, saliva droplets	2–5 months	Cirrhosis, death
Hepatitis C (epidemic form)	Viruses not precisely identified	Faeco-oral	Variable	Usually full recovery
Hepatitis C (parenteral form)	Virus not precisely identified	Parenteral (saliva in some experiments)	Variable	Death, primary hepatocellular carcinous
Herpes simplex type I	Herpes simplex virus type I	Saliva, blood contact, droplets	3–15 days	Herpetic whitlows, cold sores, post-herpetic neuralgia
Herpes simplex type II	Herpes simplex virus type II	Blood, saliva, close contact	8–14 days	Carrier state
Infectious mononucleosis	Epstein-Barr virus	Saliva, blood, close contact	5–30 days	Depression

Disease	Organism	Transmission	Incubation	Consequences
Hand, foot, mouth disease	Mainly coxsackie A16	Close contact	3–5 days	Usually none
Influenza	Influenza A and B viruses	Saliva, droplets	1–4 days	Sometimes fatal
Measles	Rubeola virus	Saliva, droplets	8–12 days	Respiratory infection, encephalopathy (rare)
Mumps	Mumps virus	Saliva, droplets	14–28 days	Sterility (men)
Bacterial				
Gonorrhoea	Neisseria gonorrhoeae	Close contact	2–10 days	Sterility, blindness
Legionellosis	Legionella	Aerosols, sprays, droplets	3–14 days	Respiratory problems, death
Staphylococcal infection	Staphylococcus aureus/ albus	Close contact	1–10 days	Boils, osteomyelitis
Syphilis	Treponema pallidum	Close contact	10–90 days	Death, CNS destruction
Tetanus	Clostridium tetani	Saliva, direct contamination, infected dentine	5–12 days	Death or disability
Tuberculosis	Mycobacterium tuberculosis	Droplets, saliva, close contact	Up to 9 months	Death or disability

of cross infection control: one for the 'high-risk' patient and one for others. The only exception to this single standard is the immunocompromised patient where there are definite reasons for taking extra precautions with special problems such as the dental-unit water supplies.

What standard of cross infection control should be adopted? The standard that is necessary is based on a knowledge of the micro-organisms, their mode of spread and preventive measures against them and their habitats. It should be simple, reproducible and its safety based on known facts.

The microbiology of cross infection control

A list of the micro-organisms which are potential sources of cross infection is shown in *Table 1.1*. Only bacteria and viruses are listed, but there is some evidence that fungi could also be involved.

Most of the micro-organisms listed in *Table 1.1* have only been *implicated* in cross infection control. The reason for this is their long incubation period and the lack of precise microbiological surveillance techniques that could prove their involvement. The long incubation period of some of the viral illnesses means that epidemiological surveys where cross infection by dentistry is suspected are often meaningless. In some instances, this is not the case and hepatitis B has been shown to be transmitted from dentists to patients.[1-4]

In all cases where infection has occurred, the cross infection procedures were inadequate. Contamination of the eye with blood has also resulted in hepatitis B transmission.[5,6] There is no doubt that hepatitis B can be transmitted by saliva and serum[7,8] and possibly from contaminated surfaces.[9] Hepatitis B is therefore an important pathogen in cross infection control.

The evidence for the transmission of other viruses is less clear. Rotaviruses and rhinoviruses can be transferred from hands to surfaces in sufficient numbers to cause human infections. It has been proved that herpes simplex type I was transmitted by a dental hygienist to patients.[10] All of these infections can be prevented by good cross infection control.[11-13]

The evidence for the transmission of HIV is more fragmentary. Unless gross blood contamination or needlestick injuries occur, then HIV is unlikely to cause infections in operative dentistry.[13,14] Such evidence is, however, unlikely to assuage the fear in patients' minds of the transmission of AIDS. Thus public concern is probably the main spur to improve standards in dentistry.

The evidence that bacteria are transmitted in dentistry is scanty. Bacteria can be transferred from instruments to patients.[15] There is circumstantial evidence that *Pseudomonas aeruginosa*[16] and *Staphylococcus aureus*[17] are also a cause of cross infection. The evidence for other micro-organisms such as *Legionella* spp. is not so firm. In the UK, the Public Health Laboratory Service has tried to establish a link between Legionnaires' disease and dentistry without any success (unpublished work).

The case for cross infection by fungi, particularly the imperfect strains, is similarly sparse. Part of this has been the lack of a suitable simple typing method. The new simple methods of identification which rely on DNA restriction methods should help resolve these questions.[18]

Risk areas

In summary, the evidence on cross infection in dentistry clearly identifies several risk areas, listed in *Table 1.2*. These can be

Table 1.2   Risk areas in dentistry

Risk area	*Preventive measure*
Hands	Gloves
Eyes	Spectacles
Direct splatter	Masks/spectacles
Aerosols	Masks
Instruments	Sterilization
Needlestick injuries	Good technique
Contaminated surfaces	Disinfection
Contaminated waste	Safe disposal/incineration

conveniently divided into personal protection, disinfection and sterilization. If these are done correctly, then cross infection control is safe for all patients.

Motivation and cross infection control

Cross infection control in dentistry will only be practised if the dentists concerned are committed to it. Recent surveys have shown that attitudes are changing rapidly: dentists are more aware of the dangers of cross infection and are implementing control in their practices.[19,20] Cross infection control needs a *team approach*, led by the dentist.

The most important part of the implementation of cross infection control is that the dentist, as head of the team, is committed to it. Without this commitment, no motivation of staff will occur.

PRACTICAL POINTS
—for staff motivation and cross infection control

- **Educate staff on microbiological aspects of dentistry**
- **Demonstrate risk areas (for example, needles)**
- **Provide regular staff training sessions**
- **Provide reinforcement and revision sessions**
- **Maintain regular procedures**
- **Correct poor technique**
- **Train *all* new staff**

2

Office design and cross infection control

Poor office design and planning make cross infection control difficult if not impossible. There are four important elements in the planning stage of an office and these are the choice of the actual room, the siting of the utilities, the space for sterilization and lastly the equipment.

Office layout

Few practices enjoy the luxury of starting from a blank piece of paper when designing an office. Usually the aim is to modify a building or suite of office space to fit the facilities required. This inevitably leads to compromise and often to mistakes.

A fundamental decision has to be made which is crucial to the overall design. The decision is whether to locate the sterilizing facilities in the office or in another part of the rooms available. If the practice has a number of dentists working in it, then the centralization of sterilizing facilities can be economic in time and in the use of space.

If a decision is made to locate the sterilizing facilities within the office, then the design is split into three distinct areas (*Figure 2.1*), which are:

- The operator's area
- The dental assistant's area
- The sterilization and storage area

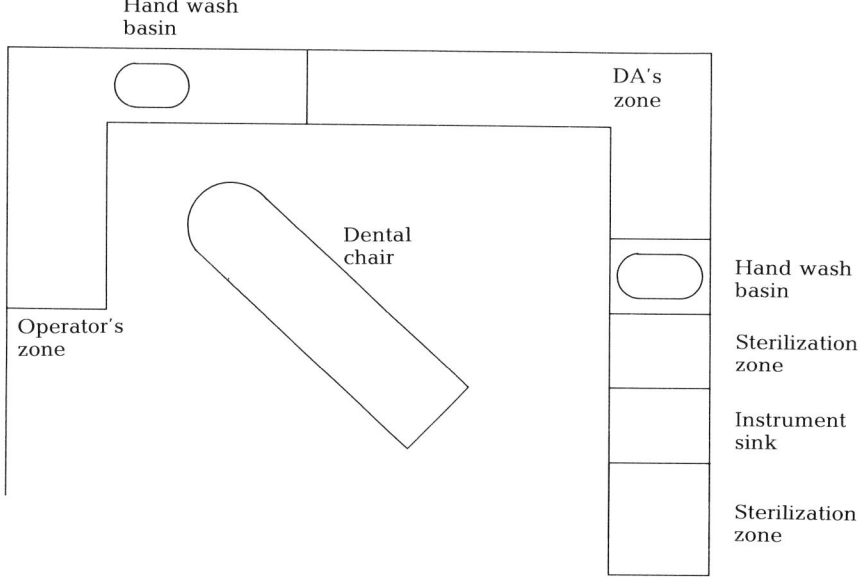

Figure 2.1　*A schematic diagram of a dental office.*

These three areas should be distinct and provided with full facilities. The operator's area can contain a sink, waste receiver and a 'dirty zone' which can be disinfected. There should also be space in a 'clean zone' for records, radiographs and documented material. The operator's zone must encompass the dental chair and ideally be predominantly sited on the side at which the patient is to enter.

The dental assistant's (DA) area will contain another dirty zone which can be disinfected together with instrument drawers and materials. It should also have a sink for hand washing and a waste receiver. This waste receiver should be larger than that for the dentist as the disposal of clinical waste will mainly be the DA's responsibility. This area will also allow easy access for the assistant to escort the patient from the surgery.

Great care should be taken to furnish the room adequately to allow for all the elements of cross infection control. Flooring should be made of material which will allow the easy treatment of spillages. Of necessity this will be some material which is impermeable and not affected by the disinfectants chosen. The use of carpet for surgery floors is not recommended. Although nowadays many carpets can be disinfected by some products, in general they are all affected deleteriously in the long term. If an office design is chosen with a consultation space and an office space, then these areas should be clearly demarcated and flooring suitable for disinfection chosen for the office space. The consultation space can of course be carpeted, with a desk and chairs for patient discussion and motivation.

It is important that the office should not be cluttered with large amounts of material and trailing wires and umbilicals for aspirators and other equipment. A design should be chosen which can be very easily cleaned by the DA and in which spillages can be easily identified and dealt with. The choice of antistatic material for flooring will tend to make the removal of dust and accumulated dirt a lot easier. Care must be taken to seal the joints between the walls and the floor with an impermeable coping to ensure that the entire floor area can be adequately cleansed. All units should allow application of disinfectant over the whole area of the cabinets and there should be no cracks or joints left for accumulation of detritus. Potted plants, flowers and other living material should not be present in the surgery as these are known to harbour pathogens and can encourage the growth of waterborne organisms. Similarly, curtains are not recommended in window spaces. The ideal are multi-slatted blinds which can be cleaned and disinfected at regular intervals by cleaning staff.

Siting of the utilities

Care must be taken to locate utilities in appropriate places. Every individual country has its own regulations for the siting of electrical supplies and compressed air facilities. These regulations must be consulted and followed precisely.

The siting of sinks is important and must be done with care. Sinks of two types are used: those for hand washing and those for cleaning instruments and disposal of liquids. It is important that sinks for hand washing are distinct from those used for cleansing instruments and they should never be mixed because of the risk of contamination. Sinks for hand washing should ideally be elbow- or foot-operated with good water-mixing devices and should be located near to towel facilities. In contrast, those for washing instruments should be deep and elbow- or foot-operated with good splash-back facilities. Sinks for cleaning or the disposal of liquid waste should ideally be large and capable of holding enough water so that if instruments are dropped they fall directly into liquid.

Space for sterilization

This space also needs careful planning and the room required is usually underestimated (*Figure 2.2*). Sterilization zones need, at the minimum, space for an ultrasonic cleaner, a deep sink with a splash-back and enough room for sterilized instruments and the sterilization device. As a rough guide, the sterilization facilities occupy at least twice as much space as the DA's area. Care should be taken when siting the sterilization device to prevent it from burning the DA. If the sterilizer generates fumes or steam, siting it next to a source of ventilation makes sense.

A central area for sterilization requires a great deal of space. A dirty area for the reception of instruments is best sited next to a sink. The ultrasonic cleaner is sited in the next area and finally the sterilization device – ideally there should be at least two such devices in case of a breakdown. Storage areas are then required and every sterilization area should have a sink for hand washing, together with space for storage of replacement materials (for example, cotton wool rolls,

Dirty area	Sink	Cleaning area	Ultra-sonic bath	Sterilizer

Figure 2.2 *A schematic diagram of the layout of a sterilization area.*

napkins). If a central sterilization facility is chosen, then it is important that this is accessible to all of the offices involved in the practice. It is also important that some simple method is devised which allows the instruments to be carried safely to the office area. Closed containers or baskets or trolleys are best used for this purpose. The central sterilization area is best sited away from the patient waiting area so that the noise of ultrasonic cleaning will not disturb the patients.

Equipment

Some care is necessary in the choice of cabinetry. Ideally all drawers and cupboards should have handles which can be easily disinfected (*Figure 2.3*). The material used to fabricate the cabinets should be suitable for disinfection treatment, both inside and outside. Butt joints where the cabinets meet the wall should be covered with a metal coping.

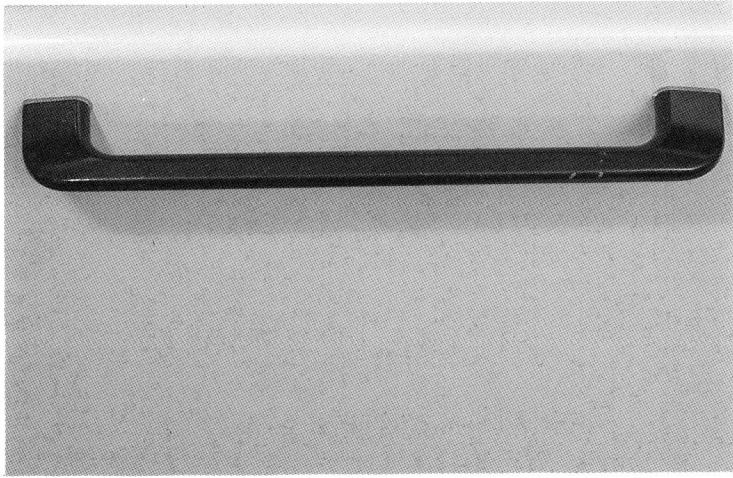

Figure 2.3 *Drawer handle that can be easily cleaned and disinfected.*

3

Personal protection

Much of the motivation for cross infection control is centred on self preservation. This self preservation is generated from fear of getting oneself infected and the medicolegal aspects and the subsequent consequences. The important elements of personal protection are avoidance of needlestick injuries, hand care, use of masks and spectacles and vaccination.

Needlestick injuries

Needlestick injuries are a potentially serious form of occupational injury in dentistry. They are defined as an injury in which contaminated material is introduced by a sharp object through the epithelium. Originally needlestick injuries were defined as being caused by needles but in dentistry they can be made by a variety of different instruments. The main risk areas are still the resheathing of local anaesthetic needles and the washing of blood-contaminated instruments. There are however other occasions when injuries can occur, good examples of which are the occasional problems when wiring fixed orthodontic appliances or the injudicious use of elevators. Needlestick injuries are serious and should be avoided at all costs.

Dentistry is perhaps the only health care profession that still practises the resheathing of needles. The reasons for this practice are valid. Even in the hand of an expert operator, the success of local analgesia, whether regional or local, is not always guaranteed. It is often necessary therefore to give additional local analgesia using the original needle and syringe. To protect the operator and staff from accidental injury, the needle is resheathed. Injuries of this kind are

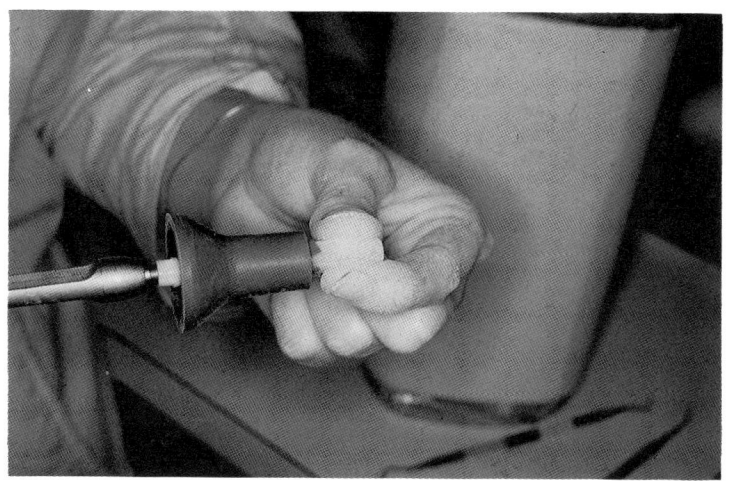

Figure 3.1a   *Non-fixed type of needleguard.*

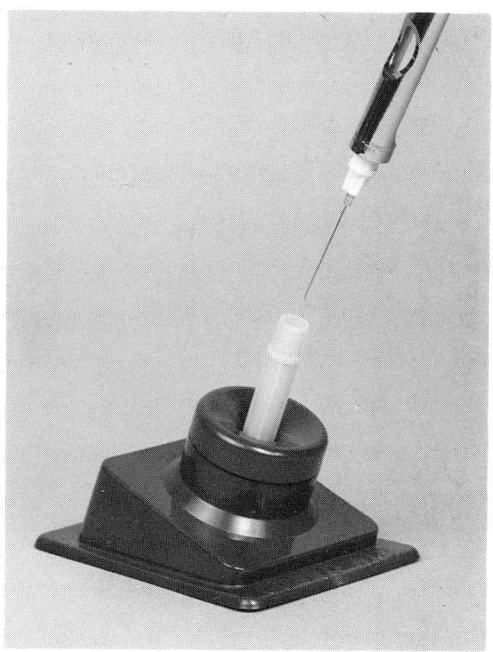

Figure 3.1b   *Fixed type of needleguard.*

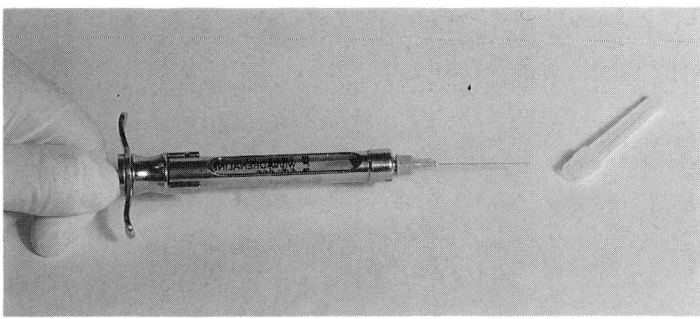

a

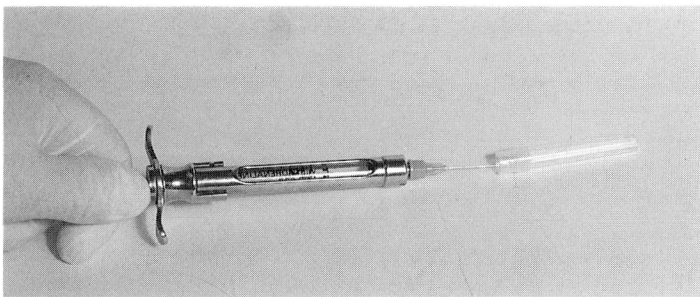

b

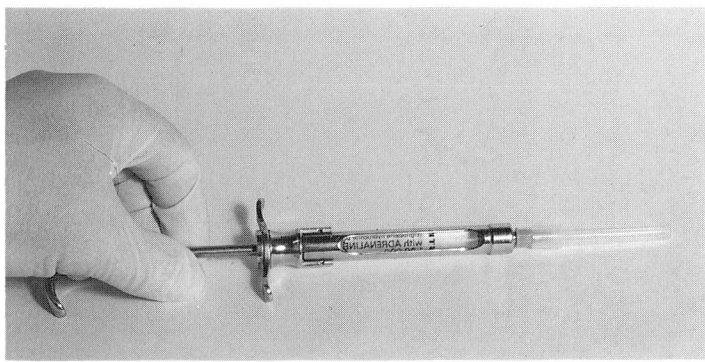

c

Figure 3.2   *The 'bayonet' method of resheathing needles*

   a   *the sheath is located one handed*

   b and **c**   *the sheath is placed over the needle and then pushed firmly into place.*

common and represent a serious health risk as potentially infectious blood can be inoculated into the operator, the most favourable situation for infection to occur. Two preventive solutions are therefore possible: the first is the use of a needleguard and the second is the 'bayonet' technique. *Figure 3.1a* and *b* shows the use of two types of needleguard, which basically guide the needle into the sheath. In the bayonet technique, the needle is introduced into the sheath one handed (*Figure 3.2*). Both of these resheathing solutions are safe and are strongly recommended.

Treatment of needlestick injuries

Needlestick injuries are potentially serious. If they occur, they must be treated in a careful manner and all members of the dental team should be aware of the procedures. The essential features of the treatment are shown in *Figure 3.3*. The immediate treatment is simple first aid. The wound should be encouraged to bleed and washed carefully under running water before it is covered with a suitable waterproof dressing.

The follow-up treatment is not so simple. Clearly the possibility of the transmission of HIV or hepatitis B virus should be considered. The use of prophylactically administered hyperimmune gammaglobulin within 10 days of inoculation has been shown to be effective in preventing hepatitis B (the gammaglobulin is obtained through a medical microbiologist or infectious-disease physician). In addition, the administration of the hepatitis B vaccine is advisable (either the serum-derived or genetically-engineered version). The question of possible HIV inoculation is again difficult. Ideally, the donor should be tested although this is not always possible as he or she may refuse. An alternative, in some cases, is to test the needle or instrument for the presence of HIV antibodies. This is often not possible as insufficient material may be present on the contaminated sharp to allow a reasonable chance for a test to be viable. It must also be remembered that HIV antibodies are not expressed continuously and a negative test result is not confirmation that HIV is absent. This quandary is difficult to resolve and expert advice from a medical microbiologist or infectious-disease physician must be sought. If there is reasonable doubt about the donor, then the use of prophylactic azothymidine should be considered. In all cases, a blood sample from the injured person should be taken and the serum from it frozen and stored. In the event of a subsequent seroconversion to an HIV

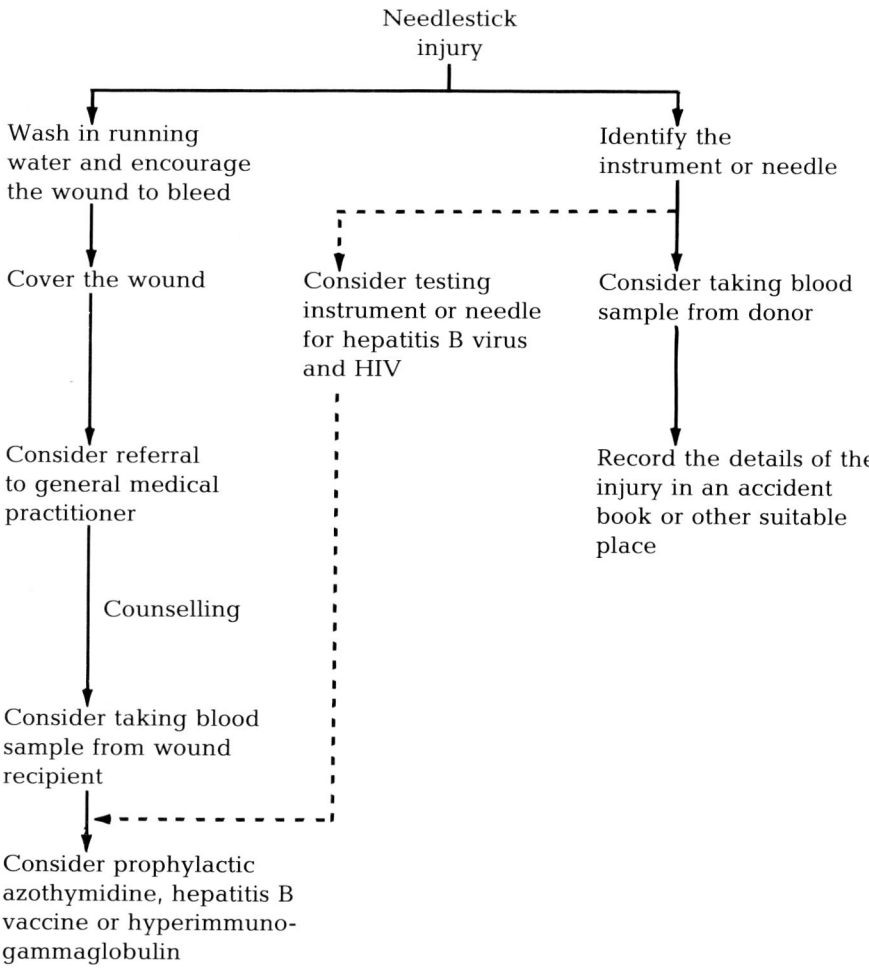

Figure 3.3 *The treatment of needlestick injury.*

antibody state, this precaution will be of considerable help in health-insurance claims or any subsequent medicolegal arguments.

The risks from needlestick injuries of transmission of HIV are not high, probably less than one per cent. The risks for hepatitis B are higher, but should be nil if all staff are vaccinated against this disease.

Hand care

Hands offer a serious risk of cross infection and should always be covered.[1,2] The risks of 'wet-fingered' dentistry are relatively high and are under discussion by some insurance and practice indemnity companies both in the UK and the USA. It is possible that in future some insurance companies may not offer full indemnity for dentists or auxiliary staff who refuse to wear gloves. Irrespective of whether gloves are worn, hand care is important if dermatological problems are to be avoided.

Dental surgeons are in the main practical people. Many engage in major hobbies of a practical nature (for example, outdoor pursuits, gardening, DIY, car maintenance). These types of hobbies are not contraindicated by a dental career but they do cause repeated minor injuries which offer a potential means for the transmission of cross infection. Any noticeable injuries (for example cuts, abrasions or other injuries) should be covered with a protective waterproof adhesive dressing before gloves are donned (*Figure 3.4*).

The rigours of practice, repeated hand washing and drying can damage the hands.[3] In particular, incomplete removal of surfactants and soaps combined with poor drying can cause the hand skin to be deleteriously affected. Complete rinsing and hand drying is essential and methods to achieve this are discussed later in this chapter. At the end of a clinical session, the use of an emollient hand cream should be a routine part of hand care. A wide variety of these creams are

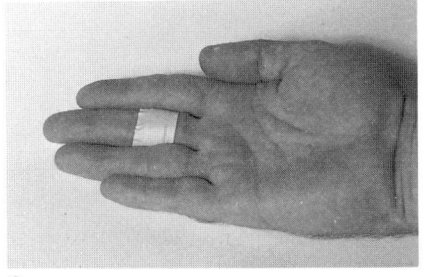
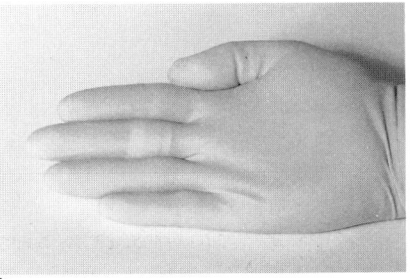

a   b

Figure 3.4   *All cuts and abrasions should be covered prior to donning of gloves.*

available and a little experimentation will yield a preparation which will keep some suppleness in the hand skin and most importantly prevent excessive drying.

A brief mention should be made about nail care. Nails should be short and reasonably manicured. Long nails break and cause problems and are unhygienic in a surgical profession.[4] Care of the nails and surrounding tissues helps to prevent paronychia.

Hand washing

Hand washing is a major part of cross infection control and should precede every clinical session. It is important for two reasons: it reduces the transient flora and it may protect the hands from infection (see the discussion on hand disinfectants later in this chapter).

The microflora of the hands can be subdivided into two types: the transient and the persistent. Transient flora is acquired from contact with contaminated objects. Most of it is rapidly lost as it cannot specifically adhere to the epithelial surfaces. Persistent flora can adhere and remain on an individual's skin. Ideally, it would be preferable to remove both the transient and persistent flora of the hands, although in practice this is almost impossible. Cross infection can arise from both types of flora. Poor hand hygiene also encourages infection from the endogenous transient and persistent hand flora.

The technique of hand washing is illustrated in *Figure 3.5*.[5] It is important that hand washing should involve every exposed aspect of the hands. At first sight, the techniques demonstrated in *Figure 3.5* look complicated, but they rapidly become routine.[6] The important point about this technique is that it covers every aspect of the hand including the finger and thumb tips, an area most at risk in surgical disciplines.

Hand washing should be performed before each session to remove transient flora and afterwards to remove any exogenously acquired flora. If gloves are worn then hand washing is necessary after they are removed, although an alcohol-based preparation may also be used.

Bar or liquid soaps?

A fundamental choice exists as to what kind of preparation to use for hand washing. The choice is between solid bar soaps or liquid

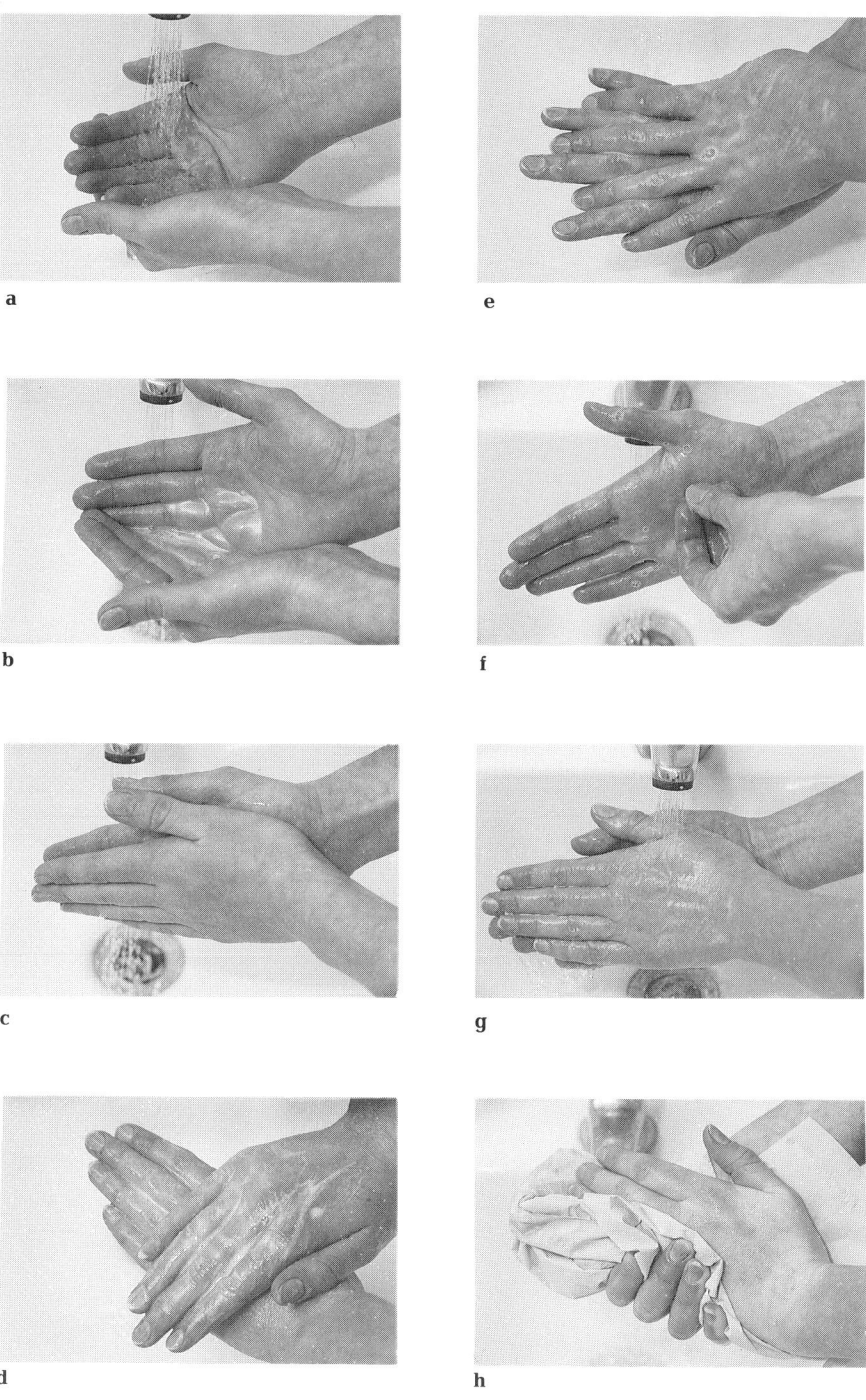

PRACTICAL POINTS
—in routine hand washing

- **Cover all cuts and abrasions**
- **Wet the hands thoroughly**
- **Use a systematic washing technique**
- **Rinse thoroughly**
- **Dry thoroughly**
- **Wash before and *after* each session**
- **Use an emollient handcream after each session**

Figure 3.5   *Hand washing procedures*

a   *Wet hands thoroughly.*

b   *Apply disinfectant.*

c   *Apply disinfectant to palms of hands.*

d   *Apply disinfectant to back of hands.*

e   *Apply disinfectant to finger webs.*

f   *Apply disinfectant to tips of fingers of both hands.*

g   *Rinse the hands thoroughly and repeat the procedure* **a** *to* **g**.

h   *Dry the hands thoroughly.*

preparations.[6] In general, bar soaps, whether medicated or not, are not recommended. They are often used by a number of different people for a multiplicity of purposes! Bar soaps can also support the growth of micro-organisms such as Staphylococci, a micro-organism strongly implicated in cross infection. Ideally, a liquid soap which combines a disinfectant should be used, as these remove a large quantity of the transient and persistent hand flora.[6]

The use of a disinfectant may also serve another important purpose. The application of a disinfectant may kill some micro-organisms but it may also impair others' pathogenicity. Initial studies with chlorhexidine preparations have shown that some Gram-negative bacteria have their pathogenicity diminished by the exposure to subcidal levels of this disinfectant.[7] The repeated use of disinfectant preparations may lead to a build up in its concentration on the hands. This may be important and protective if naked hands are exposed to infectious agents.[8]

Alcohol-based hand disinfectants

A number of hand preparations are now available which combine alcohols of various sorts and a disinfectant. The principle behind these preparations is that they combine the antimicrobial properties of a disinfectant with those of the alcohols. The desiccant action of alcohols as they evaporate from hand surfaces together with their inherent antimicrobial properties produce a strong disinfectant effect.[9] The evaporation of the alcohol leaves a residue of disinfectant on the hand. These alcohol-based preparations are applied by the same systematic method as hand-washing preparations and are very effective. The manufacturers of such products claim that they are to be used when a full hand wash is not indicated, that is when the hands are not 'soiled'. In dentistry, it is often difficult to decide when the hands are not soiled. Certainly these preparations can be used when gloves are changed if no gross contamination of the hands due to glove wearing is seen or suspected. The alcohol-based preparations are effective for disinfecting non-sterile gloves immediately before use.[10]

Alcohol-based preparations, by their very nature, do dry the skin and it is important to use an emollient hand cream at the end of the session.[3] It is possible that preparations containing disinfectants which are absorbed may give systemic effects if used in the long term. At present there is no evidence that this is important, but more research is necessary in this area.

PRACTICAL POINTS
—for the use of alcohol-based preparations

- Cover all cuts and abrasions before use
- Use in the systematic method as other hand-washing agents (*Figure 3.4*)
- Allow time for the alcohol to evaporate
- Do not use if the hand is visibly soiled with blood or saliva
- Do not use in the presence of naked flames
- Use an emollient handcream at the end of the clinical session

Eye protection

Eyes are susceptible to cross infection although the incidence of transmission by this route is unknown.[11] The vectors of this infection are most probably large particles ejected from the mouth which cause trauma and subsequent infection. The ejection of large aqueous particles may also cause cross infection. There is little evidence that fine aerosols cause similar problems. Thus eye protection, particularly against direct trauma, should always be worn for operative procedures. The principal area that needs protection is the direct line from mouth to eye. In practice, therefore, well-fitting glasses, without side-pieces, which cover the eye are satisfactory (*Figure 3.6a*). If side-pieces are comfortable, then they will add to the protection (*Figure 3.6b*).

Non-corrective and corrective spectacles and their lenses become heavily contaminated during operative procedures. Some operators choose to wash and sterilize spectacles. This is probably not necessary – careful washing with a soft tooth brush and soap to remove all particulate matter, followed by the use of a mild disinfectant, is all that is necessary.

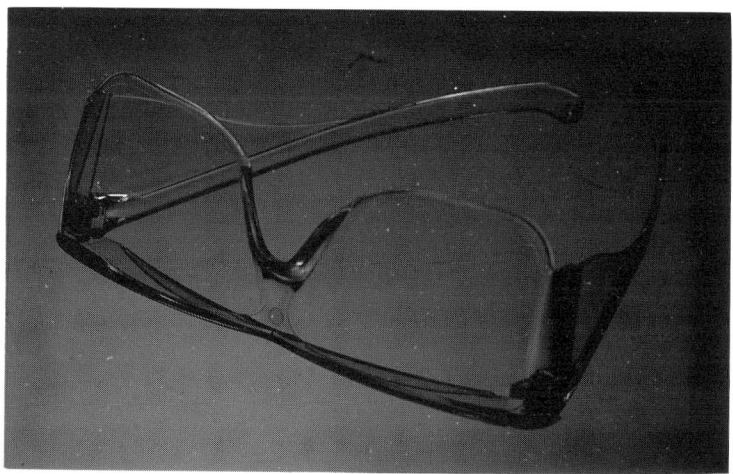

Figure 3.6a   *Simple protective spectacles.*

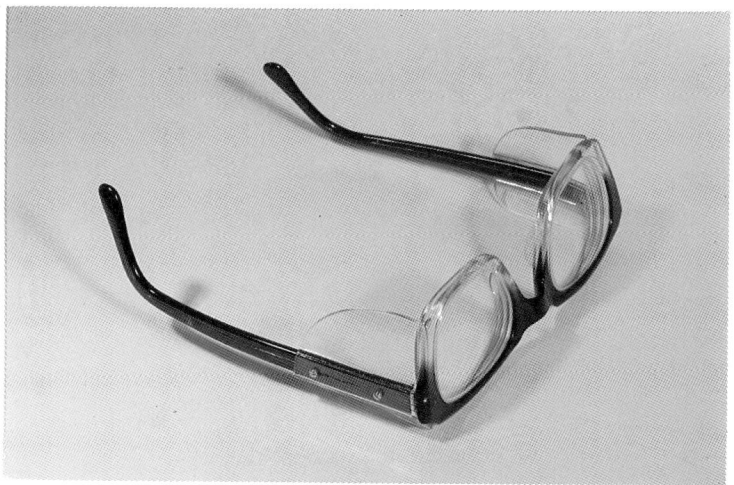

Figure 3.6b   *Corrective spectacles with side-pieces.*

Masks

The routine wearing of masks provides protection against essentially physical rather than microbiological contamination. It has been shown in a number of studies that simple masks rapidly become wet during dental procedures and consequently porous to micro-organisms.[12,13] Undoubtedly, some bacteria can penetrate wet masks, but whether these can cause infection is still not resolved.[14] Masks prevent direct 'splatter' from entering the mouth or nose. Several types of mask are available.

Simple paper masks can offer limited physical protection as they fit poorly (*Figure 3.7*). Theatre-type masks (*Figure 3.8*) are a better physical form of protection as they fit the face but they are not much of a microbiological barrier, especially when wet. They do prevent, to some extent, direct spread of droplets from the operator on to the patient. For this reason they should always be worn for elective oral surgery.[14]

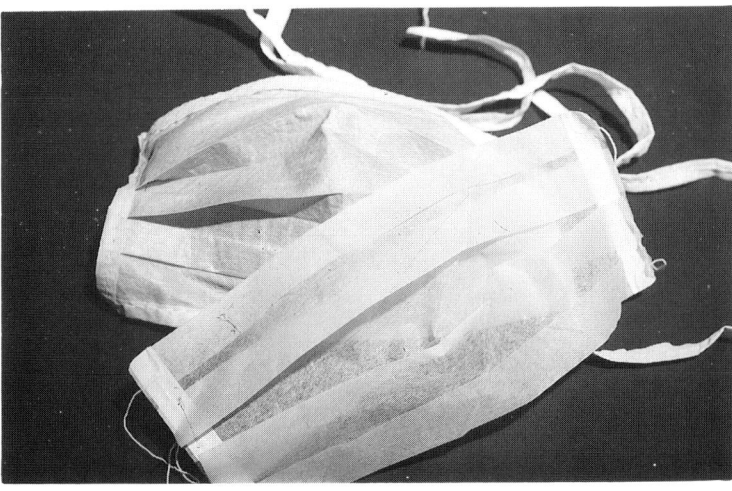

Figure 3.7 *Simple paper mask.*

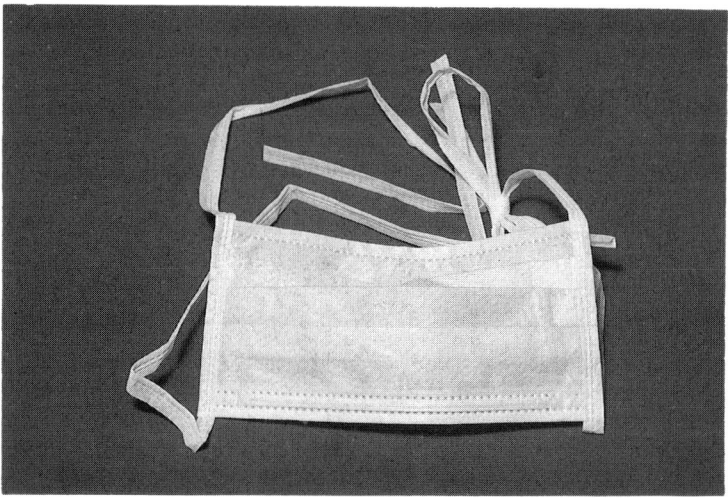

Figure 3.8   *Theatre-type mask.*

Dome-type masks are a third kind of mask, made of corrugated or laminated stiff cardboard (*Figure 3.9*). These tend to enclose the mouth and nose completely and can be hot to wear for prolonged periods. The microbiological efficacy of these masks is as yet unproven.

A more bizarre type of face protection has recently been introduced into the dental market. This consists of a full face mask of a visor type connected to an air-filtration system and pump. Air is filtered and then pumped down through a face mask. The positive pressure and unidirectional flow ensure that no infected particles are ingested. Although such a device may be interesting, in practice it is not justified as the infection risk is not proven. Such devices are also cumbersome and not ideal for the apprehensive dental patient.

Masks do become extensively contaminated and it is better that they are discarded frequently.[13] It is important to note that they are contaminated waste and should be treated appropriately.

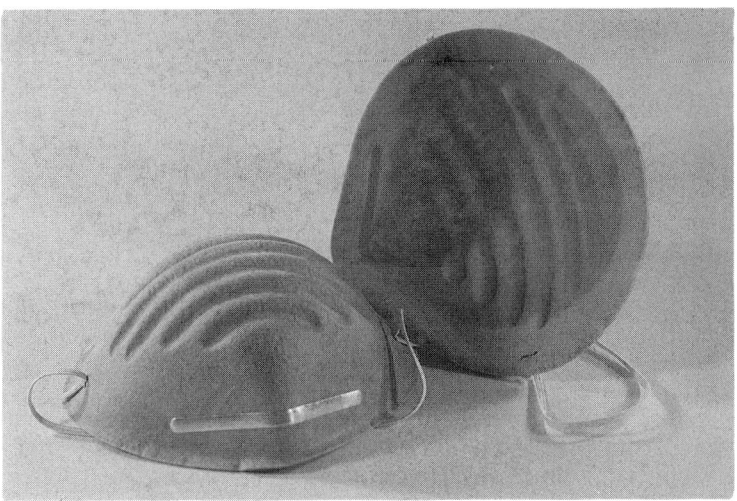

Figure 3.9   *Dome-type mask.*

PRACTICAL POINTS
—of mask wearing

- Always choose a theatre-type or well-fitting mask
- Make sure before starting work that it will adapt to the face
- Discard the mask as soon as it becomes externally contaminated
- Do not reuse masks or pull them down on to neck

Office coats, trousers and hats

There is a marked paucity of literature linking cross infection to dental office coats. Coats are in fact a simple form of protection against splatter and spillages. Ideally, office coats should be side fastening with long sleeves elasticated at the cuffs. The reason why long sleeves are recommended is that naked arms can be directly contaminated by blood or saliva. In exceptional cases, this type of contamination can lead to cross infection. Such coats may be uncomfortable to wear unless they are of light material. Coats worn for general dentistry should be frequently changed, but this is for simple personal hygiene and aesthetic reasons rather than cross infection. If a coat becomes blood contaminated it should be changed.

The wearing of operating-theatre-type hats for dentistry is not indicated, but care should be taken to ensure that hair does not interfere with vision or encroach on the surgical area. The need for white trousers and shoes is also not proven in dental cross infection control. Many operators feel that distinctive uniforms are appropriate to their practices and choose to wear them for these reasons.

Gloves

The use of operating gloves is an essential part of cross infection control. Gloves cover the body surfaces most at risk in dentistry and are highly protective. Despite all the logical, scientifically-based arguments about their efficacy, dentists in some countries still refuse to wear them. The reasons for their rejection include unfavourable patient reaction, poor fit, development of a tacky surface, loss of tactile sensitivity and damage to the hands.

Patient reaction to gloves is often overstated. In general, apprehensive patients do not tend to notice them. The apparent problem of glove sensitivity has been studied in paediatric patients and found not to be a barrier to treatment.[15] It has been this author's experience that if the reasons for glove wearing are carefully explained to patients, then any problems tend to disappear.

Poor fit of gloves is a problem. Many gloves are made to an average size and hence digit length, palm width and total volume are often at variance with biological measurements. This problem is compounded by the fact that many glove manufacturers use hand formers which were based on the dimensions of hands measured 20 years ago. This

PRACTICAL POINTS
—essentials of glove use

- **Wash hands before donning gloves**
- **Choose a glove that fits**
- **Replace glove immediately if torn**
- **Ensure chairside assistants wear gloves**
- **Wash hands immediately after glove removal**
- **Treat gloves as surgical waste and dispose of them accordingly**

leads to poor fit. The use of gloves that fit poorly compounds the problems of tactile sensitivity.

Again, it has been this author's experience that tactile sensitivity is not lost if a little care is taken in the choice of gloves. A wide range of 'dedicated' and 'examination' type gloves are now available and obtaining one that is acceptable is a matter of trial and error.[16]

Operating gloves and skin problems

A number of skin problems are associated with the wearing of gloves.[3] In practice, these are not due to glove wearing but to poor hand care. Gloves of the type used in dentistry are made from either plastic (for example, polyvinyl) or rubber (latex). True allergy to either of these agents is extremely rare. In addition to the two basic types of operating gloves there are also special types of gloves called 'low allergy' or 'hypoallergenic', and glove liners specifically designed to prevent contact of glove and skin.

Skin problems caused by gloves are usually due to dermatitis of three types: irritant contact dermatitis, allergic contact dermatitis and contact urticaria.[3]

Irritant contact dermatitis

Irritant contact dermatitis (ICD) is an inflammatory condition caused by direct damage to the skin (*Table 3.1*). It is usually associated with accumulation of irritant chemicals under a ring or other pieces of jewellery not removed before washing. It can be associated with hyperhidrosis (excessive sweating) and this is alleviated by the nightly application of 20 per cent (w/v) aluminium chloride hexahydrate in ethanol, which is then washed off in the morning.

In cases of ICD associated with atopic predisposing conditions, a dermatologist's advice should be sought. Treatment in these cases involves good hand care and the use of topical corticosteroids.

Table 3.1   Essential features of irritant contact dermatitis

Clinical features	Inflammation, blistering at point of contact
Causes	Chemical irritation
	Sweating
	Improper drying of hands
	Wearing of rings or tight-fitting jewellery
Predisposing factors	
Usual	Friction
	Occlusion (covering of surfaces)
	Sweating
Atopic	Eczema
	Asthma
	Hay fever
Cure	Avoid hand washing in very hot water
	Careful drying
	Use of emollient cream
	Frequent removal of gloves
	Hand protection for gardening and DIY tasks

Allergic contact dermatitis

Allergic contact dermatitis (ACD) is a true immunological reaction due to a hypersensitivity (type IV) reaction to glove materials. The cause of ACD is usually the accelerators, or vulcanizers, put into glove products. Amongst the specific chemicals that cause ACD are mercaptobenzothiazoles, thiurams, dithiocarbonates and guanides. ACD starts in the area covered by the gloves as an erythematous, inflammatory reaction which persists when the gloves are removed. Patch tests are needed to confirm the diagnosis. Often this type of allergy is not cured by wearing 'hypo-allergenic' or 'low-allergy' gloves as cross-reaction to chemicals contained in these can occur. Treatment is usually the removal of the allergen and the use of topical steroids. The precise type of treatment that will alleviate this problem does vary and expert advice should always be obtained.

Contact urticaria

Contact urticaria (CU) is a serious and very rare type of reaction to glove-wearing. It is an immediate-type hypersensitivity, which occurs as soon as the gloves are worn. Usually the signs of CU are local but they may take a few hours to resolve. In extreme cases, tachycardia, general urticaria and bronchospasm have been reported. The future avoidance of contact with the gloves that caused the reaction is imperative. Expert dermatological advice is mandatory. This condition is very rare.

Sterile, single-use or rewashable gloves?

The routine wearing of gloves by dentists and their auxiliary staff has given rise to a controversy about whether or not gloves should be reused.[10] The main features of the arguments for sterile, single-use or rewashable gloves are summarized in *Table 3.2*. Undoubtedly the ideal glove is one that is sterile and thrown away after use. These types of gloves should always be used for elective oral surgery procedures. In general, these gloves fit well and are expensive.

Since much of dental surgery is done in general practice where economic considerations are important, then often cheaper gloves are used. These tend to be less well fitting and hence tactile sensation may be lost. A compromise to this problem is to use a glove designed

Table 3.2   Sterile, single-use or rewashable gloves: a summary of arguments

	For	*Against*
Sterile	Ideal Well-fitting Mandatory for all oral surgery	Expensive
Single use	Cheap No possibility of cross infection	Often poorly fitting Easily torn Difficult to do delicate procedures due to lack of tactile sensation May give rise to irritant contact dermatitis
Rewashable	Economical Allow a more expensive type of glove to be used Easy to wash	Possibility of residual contamination Possibility of cross infection Cannot be reused after an HIV-antibody-positive patient May precipitate skin irritation due to excessively long wearing times

for dentistry (a 'dedicated' glove) and to rewash or disinfect it between patients. Some countries, particularly the USA, recommend that gloves are used for only *one* patient. Gloves, even if they are corrugated or dimpled for grip, are easier to wash and to remove transient flora from than hands. In practice, the majority of gloves have practically no persistent flora that cannot be removed by washing. Studies on the rewashing of gloves have shown that bacterial and viral contamination is easily removed from gloves by washing.[10,17] Gloves do deteriorate after washing and eventually become porous. The rate-limiting factor in their reuse is not, however, microbiological but physical deterioration of their surface, which causes stickiness. The physical manifestation of this problem is literally the inability to separate the fingers!

Gloves are best washed initially with alcohol-based preparations. The essential points of their use are summarized on page 33. Those strongly against glove washing dismiss the economic arguments and raise a further emotive series of questions. These questions relate to the rewashing of a glove which has been used on an HIV-antibody-positive patient and whether transfer is possible. In practice, such arguments are spurious as HIV is not known to be transmitted by this route. In real terms the emotive argument may outweigh the science.

One other problem is associated with glove-wearing and this is the inhibition of set of polyvinylsiloxane and other impression materials. In practice, most latex gloves affect the set of these materials. It is a wise precaution to check that the gloves used are compatible with the impression material. The manufacturers of the material will advise on this.

Vaccination

An important aspect of personal protection that is often overlooked by the dental team is vaccination. The list of both minor and serious illnesses that can be prevented by vaccines is large. Many dental personnel will have had some residual protection from the common illnesses as a result of childhood immunization programmes. The advent of dentistry brings new risks to any individual and these must be considered and protected against. For dental personnel, four vaccinations are important and these are against tetanus, poliomyelitis, tuberculosis and hepatitis B. The recommended schedule for vaccinations is shown in *Table 3.3*, but some explanation of the particular choice of these diseases is necessary.

Tetanus is a rare but devastating disease caused by *Clostridium tetani*. The spores of *C. tetani* are highly resistant to common disinfectants and are present in carious dentine and occasionally in dental plaque. Accidental inoculation is possible during dental procedures and, although the risk of infection is small, it is needless to take such a risk.

Mycobacterium tuberculosis is often present in saliva, as tuberculosis is still endemic in world populations. *M. tuberculosis* is a true pathogen with a low minimum infective dose. An effective vaccine prevents its transmission in dentistry.

Despite the fact that an effective, cheap, safe and easily administered oral vaccine has been available for many years, sporadic outbreaks of poliomyelitis still occur in Western civilizations. Perhaps

Table 3.3   Recommended vaccination schedule for dental personnel

	Timing and route	*Length of protection*
Tetanus	i.m.	5 years
Poliomyelitis	Oral	5 years
Hepatitis B	i.m., 0, 1, 6 months	3–5 years
Tuberculosis	Subdermal	Retest after 5 years

the reason for this is complacency. Many health-care professionals tacitly assume that poliomyelitis is no longer a problem – it is, and must be prevented. Poliomyelitis is spread by droplet infection and therefore is a real risk to dental personnel.

The viral infection hepatitis B is endemic in the world's populations and is known to be transmitted by saliva and blood. Vaccines are now available in two principal forms. The serum-derived preparation is purified hepatitis B surface antigen (HBsAg, sometimes called the Australia antigen) from the serum of blood donors who have had the disease. Since many of the donors were of unknown disease status, it was originally believed that this vaccine was contaminated with HIV. This is in fact not the case, as the vaccine purification process prevents this being even a remote possibility. The Centers for Disease Control in the USA investigated the possibility of the serum-derived vaccine being contaminated and unequivocally pronounced it safe.

The other form of the vaccine is a genetically engineered preparation. The part of the DNA genome that encodes for hepatitis B surface antigen has been identified and sequenced. The sequence has been transferred by an appropriate vector into the brewer's yeast *Saccharomyces cerivisiae*. This transformed yeast is grown and it produces the surface antigen which is purified. This is appropriately diluted and used for vaccination. Clearly, since no serum products are involved, there is no possibility of other infections being present. Ironically some of the proteins from the yeast may be present in the vaccine and these may very occasionally cause side-effects.

The efficacy of the two hepatitis B vaccines is high, greater than 95 per cent in both cases. It is difficult to be dogmatic as to how long protection is maintained; however 3 to 5 years' immunity is thought to be conferred. The rate of seroconversion is between 95 and 99 per cent. Studies have shown that some vaccine recipients apparently do not seroconvert or have low serum antibody levels. For this reason, some centres recommend routine serum testing for circulating anti-HBsAg antibodies. This has led in some cases, where antibody levels have been low, to multiple booster vaccinations. It is difficult to assess whether such multiple boosters are necessary. Over one million courses of the vaccine have been given, many to high-risk groups, without any single incidence of subsequently acquired hepatitis B infection. The antibody status of the vast majority of these recipients has not been known and it follows that many may have had low circulating levels, but still had protection. What probably matters is not circulating antibody titres but immunological memory; at present no simple, safe challenge test is available to assess this properly. It is therefore best at present to follow a physician's advice on this matter.

Individual countries have different problems with endemic infectious disease and it is therefore best to obtain and follow the recommended vaccination policies for the prevention of infectious disease.

It would be remiss not to mention rubella before leaving the subject of vaccines. Approximately 15 per cent of women do not experience rubella infection before child-bearing age is reached. Rubella is a known teratogen and can cause congenital malformations of the foetus, particularly in the first trimester of pregnancy. It could be transferred by dental procedures and so it is desirable that, before any clinical work is undertaken, female dentists intending to have children are vaccinated against rubella.

4

Sterilization

Sterilization is the killing of all micro-organisms whether vegetative or pathogenic. Sterilization is described as an absolute term as it is very difficult to maintain. Sterilization is best reserved for those instruments which become contaminated with blood and saliva and are involved with breaches in the epithelium. Sterilization of an instrument can only be achieved if three definite stages are completed,[1] these are:

- presterilization cleaning
- the sterilization process
- aseptic storage

Presterilization cleaning

The object of sterilization is to denature the micro-organisms and hence to render them non-viable. In order to kill the micro-organisms, they must be accessible and not covered in organic detritus. If organisms are covered in organic matter then it is possible for them to be insulated from the sterilization process and to remain viable. Presterilization cleaning is an essential step and should be done carefully and thoroughly. There are three methods that can be used: manual, ultrasonic or mechanical washing; some machines combine the latter two methods.

Manual cleaning

Manual cleaning is the simplest and cheapest method of presterilization. It is, however, time-consuming and may be difficult to achieve.
Clearly the end result of manual cleaning depends on the assiduous-
ness and application of the operator. One prerequisite is that heavy-
duty gloves must be worn, as needlestick injuries are common in this
process, and glasses must be worn to protect the eyes. Many of the
instruments (for example burs) require a lot of patience if thorough
cleaning is to be achieved. When manual cleaning is being undertaken, it is best done in a deep sink partially filled with water. The
water is useful to prevent damage if the instrument is accidentally
dropped. The use of a liquid detergent helps the cleaning process. In
the author's opinion, manual cleaning is best reserved for removing
residual material from instruments after some other mechanical
method has been used.

Ultrasonic cleaning

Ultrasonic cleaning relies on agitation of the instrument and hence
the liquid surrounding it, so that material is removed from the surface.
It is perhaps the most frequently used method of presterilization
cleaning, and yet its effects on micro-organisms have not been
completely studied. At present, it is not known what is the best liquid
to use in an ultrasonic bath, nor the optimal time for cleaning. There
is no doubt that, for small instruments with complicated surfaces, such
as burs, ultrasonic cleaning is the method of choice. However,
ultrasonic agitation can damage instruments and burs in particular
can lose their edge.[2] Burs and other small instruments are best put in
some form of small container (*Figure 4.1*), such as a plastic beaker, to
prevent them being lost in the base of the ultrasonic cleaner.

   Whatever liquid is used in the ultrasonic cleaner, it is best to change
it regularly (at least once every day). Many of the recommended
ultrasonic bath solutions contain disinfectants and these are rapidly
inactivated by the released proteinaceous matter. There is some
evidence that ultrasonic cleaning may kill some viruses, but this may
depend on the amount of protein present.[3] It is also dependent upon
the time in the ultrasonic bath and what solution is used. This author
has used an ultrasonic cleaning time of approximately two minutes
with good results. However, the time required is that which gets the
instrument clean.

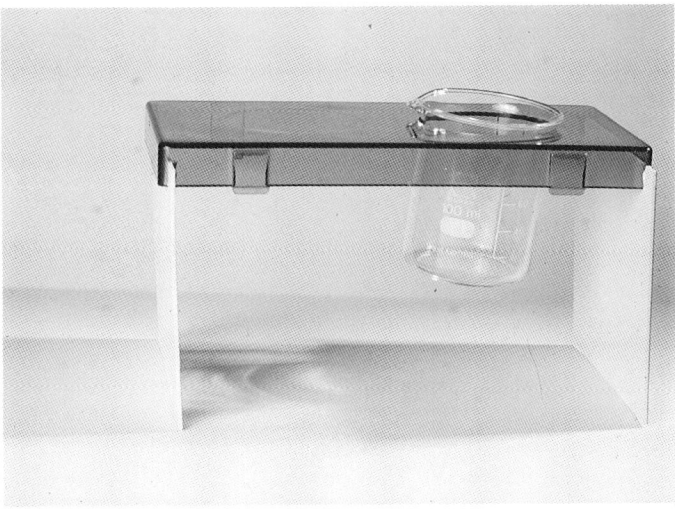

Figure 4.1   *Burs are best put into a small container before being placed in an ultrasonic bath.*

Ultrasonic baths do make a lot of noise which can be disturbing to some patients. Their location and use in an office whilst a patient is being treated can cause distress. The noise of an ultrasonic cleaner can be considerably reduced if a cover is employed when it is in use.

Mechanical washing

Mechanical washing is used extensively in Europe and is an effective method of presterilization cleaning. It works on the dishwasher principle, by squirting high-pressure jets of water with or without a detergent. The only disadvantage to mechanical washing is that it is time-consuming and small items such as burs are not suitable for use in all machines.

Ultrasonic and mechanical cleaning

A combination of ultrasonic and mechanical cleaning is used in some machines. These tend to be expensive and more suitable for hospital sterile supplies departments. They are by far the most efficient method of achieving presterilization cleaning.

Presterilization check

Whatever method is chosen for presterilization cleaning, it is important that it is followed by a manual check. If any residual detritus is noticed, it must be removed.

Sterilization process

Theoretically, there are at least five methods to sterilize dental instruments:

- boiling water
- chemicals
- dry heat
- autoclaves
- chemiclaves

Boiling water

Boiling water has been extensively used for killing micro-organisms for many decades. Micro-organisms can be killed by exposure to boiling water if the time period is long enough. The killing process takes an inconveniently long time (up to one day for some micro-organisms).[4] Clean water must also be used for every cycle and a temperature of 100°C must be maintained. In practice, this is not how boilers are used;[5] the water is not changed and is often contaminated, the boiler does not reach 100°C and the length of the cycle is dependent on the operator. They are not recommended for use in dental practice as they are an unreliable method for instrument sterilization.

Chemicals

Chemicals can be used to sterilize instruments. The common ones used are the aldehydes, gluteraldehyde or formaldehyde. In hospital practice, ethylene oxide has been used for many years; the expense of the plant necessary precludes its routine use in dental practice. Gluteraldehyde and formaldehyde are very effective in the destruction of micro-organisms but the process takes time. For any instrument, presterilization cleaning must be satisfactorily completed.

The period of immersion for sterilization is a matter of some controversy. Some authorities recommend a multi-stage technique (*Figure 4.1*), others a single long period of immersion. What is not controversial is that the whole process of immersion is lengthy and must not be disturbed by the immersion of more instruments.

The sterilization chemicals are highly irritant and must be aseptically rinsed from the instruments with sterile water. In addition, after this has been completed, the instruments must be aseptically stored. This is a complicated and difficult process and is not easily and satisfactorily achieved in dental practice. In recent surveys, dipping

PRACTICAL POINTS
—scheme for sterilization of dental instruments in gluteraldehyde

- **Immerse instruments in *fresh* 2 per cent (w/v) gluteraldehyde for 1 hour**
- **Reimmerse in *fresh* 2 per cent (w/v) gluteraldehyde for 3 hours**
- **Wash with sterile water**
- **Dry aseptically**
- **Store in a sterile dry container**

techniques of indeterminate lengths have been shown to be widely used by dental practitioners.[6] This practice is dangerous and is not to be recommended.

One other problem is associated with the use of chemical sterilization solutions; this is their inherent irritancy. Aldehydes can cause respiratory problems, contact dermatitis and be irritant to the eyes. Protective spectacles, heavy-duty gloves and an apron are recommended during the use of these chemicals. This is probably not enough, however, as some countries are now questioning any use of such chemicals. In the UK, the permitted exposure limits to aldehydes have recently been defined (COSH regulations). These exposure levels are very low and almost preclude the use of these chemicals for routine sterilization. There is also a question as to whether these chemicals are carcinogenic.

Dry heat

Dry heat is a simple method of instrument sterilization. It does, however, have severe disadvantages. The recommended temperature and time combinations are 180°C for 30 minutes and 160°C for one hour. These are the *holding* times and do not include any warming-up or cooling-down periods. In practice, the time taken to sterilize an instrument at 180°C is in excess of 90 minutes as cooling down tends to be prolonged. The cycle of most hot-air ovens can be interrupted and this can prevent sterilization.

One serious drawback to hot-air oven use is the presence of 'cool' spots. In the simple type of hot-air ovens, the temperature can vary quite considerably in various parts of the oven particularly if loading is not carefully done. Circulation fans, fitted to the more sophisticated ovens, improve the temperature differentials, but often do not cure the problem. Hot-air ovens also char most cotton materials and temper instruments. With present designs, hot-air ovens are not recommended for sterilization in dental practice unless fitted with a time lock and adequately controlled by thermocouples.

Autoclaves

The autoclave is a machine which sterilizes by using steam under pressure. Most of its cidal action is thought to be by a process of denaturation, but oxidation undoubtedly occurs as well. What is important in the autoclave is the latent heat carried by steam under pressure. Although the moisture in the steam helps, it is this heat which kills the micro-organisms.

Autoclaving can fail if the machine is not loaded properly to ensure free circulation of steam and heat. Thus it is possible to trap pockets of air in autoclaves which insulate the items to be sterilized. In sophisticated vacuum autoclaves, the air is removed by an evacuation pump. These autoclaves are expensive and time consuming to operate and are not often used in dental practice. Non-vacuum autoclaves use the incoming steam pressure to evacuate the air. The design of non-vacuum autoclaves has improved to such an extent that modern ones are almost as efficient in air removal as the vacuum type. Thus it is unusual to trap significant amounts of air in autoclaves. Of course this can be achieved if the autoclave is overloaded. A good working rule is to check that the autoclave is loaded to ensure free circulation of steam around the items to be sterilized. Most modern autoclaves have indwelling temperature sensors (thermocouples) linked to microprocessors which automatically ensure that the correct amount of heat is delivered to the load.

The temperature and time combination for autoclaves is shown in *Table 4.1*. Autoclaves are an efficient way of sterilizing instruments but they do have some disadvantages. The two principal disadvantages are rusting of instruments and their wetness after the process has finished. The rusting of instruments is an almost insoluble problem. Various agents such as 0.1 per cent (w/v) sodium nitrate can be used to ameliorate the problem but they leave residues which are difficult to remove. The wetness of the instruments can be avoided by the purchase of an autoclave with a drying cycle.

Table 4.1   Temperature and time combinations for autoclaves

Temperature (°C)	Minimum hold time (mins)
134–138	3
126–129	10
121–124	15
115–118	30

Chemiclaves

Chemical vapour sterilization (CVS) is based on a mixture of water, formaldehyde, acetone, methyl ethyl ketone, ethyl alcohol, methyl alcohol, tertiary butyl alcohol and isopropyl alcohol. This mixture is allowed to penetrate the load and held at a temperature of 132°C for 20 minutes. The great advantage of this machine is that, unlike the autoclave, it will not rust metal instruments and it is therefore ideal for delicate ones. The vapours used in this machine can be toxic and need to be removed effectively once the process is completed. This is done by a 'scavenger' device, a type of filter which absorbs the vapours.

Chemical vapour sterilization is extensively used in the USA and some parts of Europe. It is particularly useful for such instruments as orthodontic pliers where rusting of the joints may cause problems. In the UK, the use of chemical vapour is not condoned in dental practice due to the potential toxicity of the vapours. There is no doubt that the

Table 4.2   The chemical vapour sterilizer and the autoclave: advantages and disadvantages

Sterilizer	*Advantages*	*Disadvantages*
Chemical vapour	Does not rust instruments	Costly to buy chemicals
	Ideal for orthodontic instruments	Needs a scavenger device
		Must be carefully maintained
		Has a long cycle
Autoclave	Cheap to run and buy	Rusts some instruments
	Useful for most instruments	Needs a drying cycle
	Can have short cycles	

removal of the vapours depends on the sterilizer being properly maintained. The chemical vapour sterilizer is expensive to use as the chemicals must be bought. *Table 4.2* summarizes the advantages and disadvantages of the autoclaves and chemical vapour sterilization processes.

Hot-bead sterilizer

Hot-bead sterilizers were designed to sterilize reamers and files that are used to clean multi-rooted pulp cavities during endodontic treatment. This prevents 'carry over' of micro-organisms between root canals and hence cross infection. The exact length of time this sterilization takes is very instrument-dependent and the manufacturer's instructions should be followed. Glass bead sterilizers should not be used for anything other than endodontic instruments.

Aseptic storage

The third part of the sterilization process is aseptic storage. It is a waste of effort to clean an instrument, sterilize it and then store it unwrapped in a drawer. The ideal way to store instruments is dry in a protective container. Fundamentally, there are two systems that are useful for aseptic storage: instrument trays and sterilization bags (often called sterilization pouches).[7]

Instrument trays come in a variety of sizes, shapes and colours (*Figure 4.2*). They can be adapted for set surgical routines. The instruments are sterilized in the trays and the lid is replaced after the process is complete. Instrument trays, when lidded, act in a similar fashion to Petri dishes. A loose but airtight lid is more than adequate for storage for periods of years without danger. Many practitioners bind these lids down with tape but this is not necessary. The important points are that the lid should fit reasonably well and that the instruments should be dry. This latter point is crucial as all biological reactions take place in water. If no water is available, then no microbial metabolism occurs. Dry storage is simple and economical.

What must be strongly deprecated is the practice of dipping or storing instruments in disinfectant after sterilization. Disinfectants (*Chapter 5*) are rapidly inactivated by protein, heat and often by light.

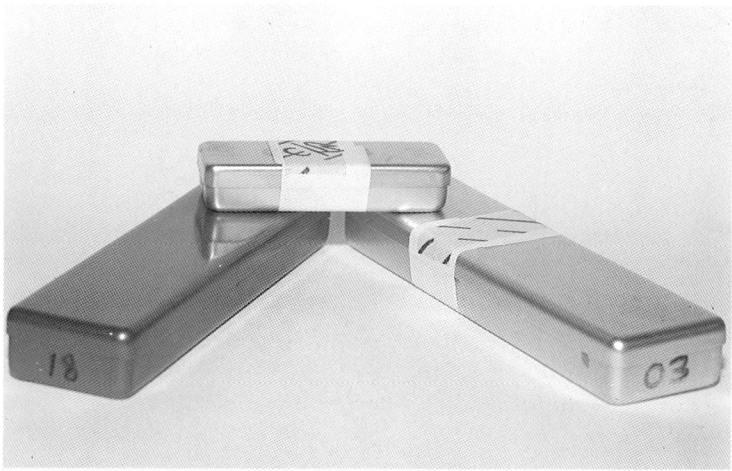

Figure 4.2 *Instrument sterilization tray and lid.*

The constant transfer of instruments into a disinfectant reduces its antimicrobial properties. In these circumstances, contamination may occur rather than disinfection.

Sterilization bags or pouches have previously only been recommended for use in vacuum autoclaves. Recent studies have shown that, provided some form of sterilization monitor is put into the bag, then this method of storage can be used in non-vacuum autoclaves (*Figure 4.3*).[7] It is important to squeeze out as much air as possible from the bag to prevent insulation of the instruments. Critics of sterilization bags have suggested that since bags are often wet following sterilization, this may cause recontamination. The mechanism for this is that micro-organisms may penetrate the bag in water. Tests carried out by this author with motile bacteria have repeatedly failed to demonstrate this phenomenon. In this author's opinion, bags are a safe and suitable method of aseptic storage for dental instruments, provided that they contain a sterilization indicator.[8] They must be stored dry. They are particularly useful for surgical instruments that are used intermittently.

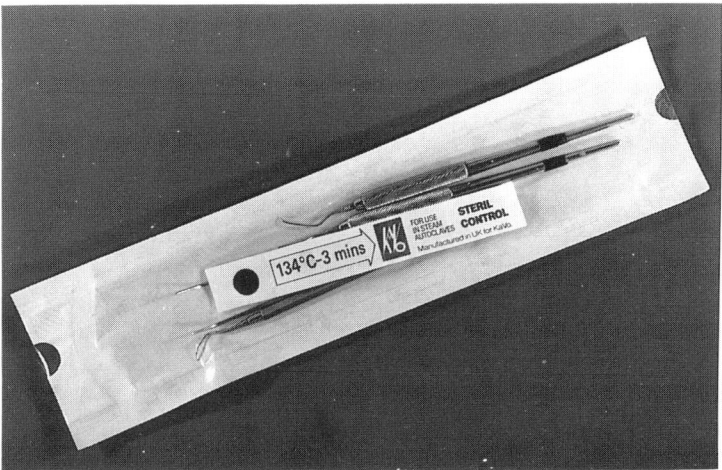

Figure 4.3 *A sterilization bag. Note the presence of the temperature steam and time strip which has changed colour to indicate satisfactory sterilization.*

Sterilization indicators

Sterilization indicators (often called process indicators) are devices which are used to determine whether sterilization has occurred. There are two sorts of indicators: biological and non-biological. Biological indicators are usually cultures of *Bacillus stearothermophilus* or *Bacillus subtilis*. *B. subtilis* test strips are usually reserved for dry-heat sterilizers and *B. stearothermophilus* for autoclaves. After use, the strips are cultured in media and any growth is indicative of sterilization failure. It is possible to obtain anomalous results with these biological indicators depending on their exact method of use. For the practitioner, the culture of these bacteria is also difficult and often inconvenient.

Non-biological sterilization indicators are usually based on physical or chemical principles. The most reliable indicator is the externally calibrated thermocouple linked to a time monitor. These thermocouples are reliable and accurate and are perhaps the ultimate test of heat-dependent sterilization processes.[5] Many autoclaves incorporate thermocouples linked to microprocessors and in general these are reliable. Annual recalibration is recommended.

A variety of chemical-based indicators are available. Autoclave tape and Brownes' tubes are indicators which show that the apparatus has reached the correct temperature; they omit the essential time element. Indicators such as TST (temperature steam and time) strips are useful for monitoring sterilization in autoclaves. These are strongly recommended (*Figure 4.4*).[8]

Sterilization should be monitored routinely by placing an indicator in the most inaccessible part of the load. In an ideal world, it would be monitored for every load, but this is often impracticable. Various recommendations have been made about the periodicity of testing by national authorities and it is recommended that these are adhered to by practitioners.

Difficult instruments

Before leaving the subject of sterilization it is important to consider the difficult instruments to sterilize. These are handpieces, burs and air and water syringe nozzles.

Handpieces

Handpieces are comparable to the scalpel handles of surgeons. They become heavily externally contaminated with blood and saliva. Handpieces do, however, become heavily internally contaminated as well by aspiration of material into the air and water lines. This is due to the positive retraction devices fitted to most dental units to prevent accidental spraying of the patient's face with water. These retraction devices result in heavy bacterial contamination which could cause cross infection. External disinfection of the handpiece is therefore not sufficient and the handpieces must be sterilized. Most handpieces can now be sterilized if they have a permissive temperature, a boiling water beaker or both stamped on them (*Figure 4.5*). Considerable controversy exists as to whether some handpieces are fully sterilizable. Since the purchase of handpieces represents a considerable capital outlay it is important that expensive non-autoclavable handpieces are excluded. It is important that high-quality oil is used for lubrication before every sterilization cycle. Sterilized handpieces may

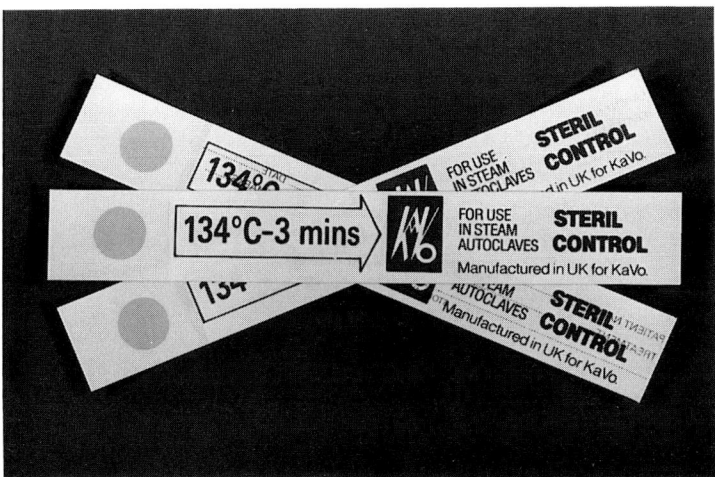

Figure 4.4   *Temperature steam and time strip. The small coloured dot on the left changes colour when sterilization is complete (for an example of the change, see Figure 4.3).*

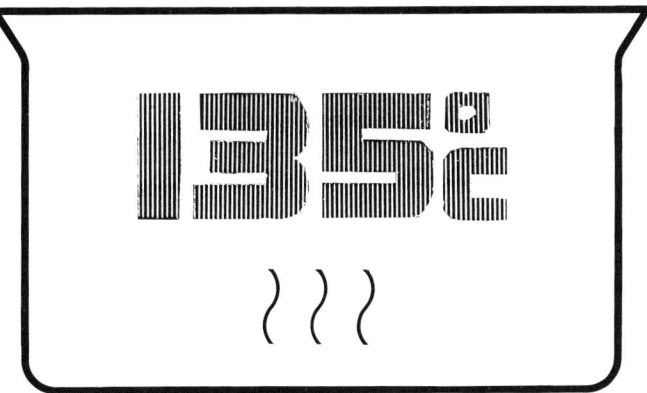

Figure 4.5   *The permissive temperature stamp on handpieces. This is stamped onto handpieces and indicates the maximum temperature to which the instrument may be heated without causing it damage.*

PRACTICAL POINTS
—in the selection of autoclavable handpieces

- **Obtain a guarantee that the handpiece is sterilizable**
- **Obtain from the manufacturer the maximum permissive temperature for handpiece sterilization and do not exceed it**
- **Use only lubricant oils recommended by the manufacturer**
- **Use oil before every sterilization cycle**
- **Clean external parts of the handpiece before sterilization**
- **Do not sterilize handpieces with burs in situ**

---

need their bearings changed more frequently than those not exposed to heat processes.

Some new designs of handpieces and units have no water-retraction mechanisms. It is argued that these do not need sterilization, only disinfection. At the present time, the evidence for this lack of sterilization is far from complete. It is safer therefore to sterilize all handpieces.

Burs

If handpieces are the equivalent of a scalpel handle, then burs are equivalent to the blade. All burs should be sterile. Steel burs do not withstand this process and therefore should be regarded as disposable. Diamond and tungsten carbide burs are deleteriously affected by sterilization and only withstand a minimum of sterilization cycles. The number is dependent on the process of manufacture. Clearly this is an area where further research is necessary.

Air and water syringe tips

There is now considerable evidence that the tips of these syringes become very contaminated before use. They do require sterilization after cleaning.

Disposables

It may seem odd to finish a chapter on sterilization with a discussion about disposables. There is a mistaken belief amongst some practitioners that disposable items such as needles can be sterilized. This is dangerous as the fine-gauge needles used in dentistry cannot be satisfactorily sterilized. Other items such as local anaesthetic cartridges should not be reused as undetected blood products are often aspirated onto them during injection. In general, disposable items are as their name suggests – disposable.

5

Disinfection, disposal of contaminated waste and decontamination

The term 'disinfection' is defined as the removal or inactivation of some micro-organisms. This definition implies that only some, not all, pathogenic micro-organisms will be removed. Many practitioners confuse disinfection with sterilization both in semantic and practical terms. In any practice, there should be a clear definition of what should be sterilized and what should be disinfected. A good working rule is that any instrument that comes routinely into contact with blood, saliva or tissues that are surgically breached should be sterilized. Any other instrument should be disinfected. Disinfection should therefore be reserved for the following:

● decontamination of surfaces

● treatment of spillages

● decontamination of areas known to be grossly contaminated

● decontamination of non-surgical instruments

● decontamination prior to sterilization

● disinfection of dental-unit water supplies

Unfortunately, many practitioners use disinfection as a substitute for sterilization; such a practice is dangerous. There has been an explosion in the number of disinfectants available for dentistry. The advertising associated with disinfectants is at times wondrous to behold and mostly bears no relation to what a disinfectant actually does in dentistry. In fact, in most situations, a disinfectant exhibits three principal properties:

- dilution of the micro-organisms present
- cleaning of the area or instrument
- a cidal or static action

Dilution of micro-organisms

A finite number of micro-organisms are usually required for an infection to be established. This number is defined as the minimum infective dose (MID). The act of putting a liquid disinfectant on a surface effectively dilutes the micro-organisms below the MID. It necessarily follows that any contamination will not usually result in an infection. This dilution principle is often ignored by clinicians but it probably is the most important part of disinfection.

Cleaning

The act of putting a disinfectant on a surface and wiping it off has a cleaning effect. This part of applying a disinfectant is important in infection control. Disinfectants are inactivated by blood or other organic detritus. Thus any cidal or static power that they possess will be severely reduced if the micro-organisms they are intended to kill are protected from their action. Cleaning must, therefore, be a part of the disinfection process.

Cidal or static action

The science associated with the use of disinfectants is very complex and is described eloquently in other texts.[1–3] In general, each disinfectant has either a cidal or a static action. The exact method of action of each disinfectant is also dependent upon:

- concentration
- contact time
- micro-organisms present

PRACTICAL POINTS
—for storage and use of disinfectants

- **Do not expose to extremes of heat or cold**
- **Do not reuse**
- **In general keep away from sunlight**
- **Dilute to manufacturer's instructions**
- **Always wear protective clothing during use**

Many disinfectants have a specific concentration that must be used if they are to work. Exceeding this concentration may cause a *fall* in the disinfectant power. A good example of this is isopropyl alcohol which has greater disinfectant action at 70 per cent (w/v) dilution than when undiluted. The manufacturer's instructions for dilution must therefore be followed every time. The contact time of the micro-organisms with the disinfectant is also critical. This is linked to disinfectant concentration and is micro-organism dependent. Various micro-organisms are therefore killed or rendered static by a variety of concentration and time combinations, according to the type of disinfectant.

Disinfection test

The testing of disinfectants and the assessment of the results form a complicated process. There are in fact a large number of available tests, all of which measure different parameters. In an attempt to try to make the tests and use of disinfectants more applicable to their properties, the US Environmental Protection Agency (EPA) set up an accreditation programme for disinfectants.[3] The disinfectants were divided into those suitable for *surfaces* and those suitable for *immersion* of instruments. The available types of disinfectants will be reviewed together with their EPA approvals.

Aldehydes

Two aldehydes have been used in dentistry: formaldehyde and gluteraldehyde. Formaldehyde is too irritant to be used routinely. Gluteraldehyde is also irritant but can be used with care – a summary of its advantages and disadvantages is shown in *Table 5.1*. It is important that skin protection is worn when the preparation is used. Gluteraldehyde at a concentration of 2 per cent (w/v) is recommended by the EPA for immersion of instruments only. Gluteraldehyde is EPA-approved for reuse, but great care must be taken not to use it for too long as it is inactivated. The best preparations are those that are buffered to an alkaline pH.

Halogen-based disinfectants

There are two halogen-based disinfectants that are EPA-approved: the iodophors and hypochlorite. The iodophors (*Table 5.2*) are safe, non-irritant disinfectants that are recommended for surface disinfection by the EPA. These preparations are best sprayed on to the surface, wiped off with paper towels and then sprayed on again. The surface can then be left to dry naturally or rewiped. If this process is repeated during the day, the amount of disinfectant on the surface accumulates and is highly effective against contamination. The iodophors are more active in aqueous solution than in alcohol. Hypochlorite has a similar action to the iodophors and is suitable for surface disinfection. Some people object to the odour of chlorine, but it is effective.

Phenols

Phenol has been used for disinfection since the time of Lister. Phenols have a pungent, penetrating odour which tends to persist on clothing. Although phenols are highly effective against most micro-organisms (*Table 5.3*), there are others that can withstand their action or even degrade them for their own metabolism. They are not recommended by the EPA for either immersion or surface disinfection. A number of phenols are manufactured for dentistry: cresols, hexachloraphene, resorcinols and chlorhexidine gluconate. The latter compound is useful for hand washing.

Table 5.1   Gluteraldehyde for instrument disinfection: advantages and disadvantages

Advantages	Disadvantages
Is effective against most pathogenic micro-organisms	Irritant
	Has an unpleasant odour
Can be used for instrument immersion	Causes contact dermatitis in some individuals
	Loses activity on storage or exposure to light
	Can cause surface changes in some instruments
	Some preparations need an activator
	Not recommended as a surface disinfectant

Table 5.2   Halogen disinfectants: advantages and disadvantages

Advantages	Disadvantages
Good surface disinfectant	Not suitable for immersion
Non-irritant	Rapidly loses activity on storage or exposure to sunlight
Action can be cumulative	
Active against a wide range of micro-organisms	
Inexpensive	

Table 5.3   Phenols for disinfection: advantages and disadvantages

Advantages	Disadvantages
Effective against some micro-organisms	Pungent odour
Effective as pretreatment mouth washes	Can be easily inactivated
Useful for hand washing	Can be degraded by some micro-organisms

Quaternary ammonium compounds

There are a number of these compounds, such as cetyl pyridium chloride, alkyl dimethyl benzylammonium chloride and mono- and dibenzalkonium chloride. All of these compounds have limited antimicrobial activity and are not recommended for dentistry.

Alcohols

Considerable debate surrounds the action of isopropyl and ethyl alcohols as disinfectants. The EPA does not recommend their sole use as either a surface or an immersion disinfectant. There are, however, contrary views to this depending on the type of tests used to evaluate them.[4] The problem with the use of these compounds is that their action is not predictable and depends on the clinical situation and type of organic material present. Alcohols are often combined with phenols or other chemicals and this action can be synergistic. The desiccant action of alcohol can also be virucidal.

Peroxygenated compounds

A class of compounds that has recently been introduced is the peroxygenated compounds. These release nascent oxygen and contain a detergent which also has antimicrobial action. They are known

Table 5.4   Summary of disinfectants

Type	Surface	Immersion
Iodophors	Yes	No
Gluteraldehyde	No	Yes
Alcohols	No	No
Alcohols and additives	Yes	No
Quaternary ammonium compounds	No	No
Peroxygenated compounds	Yes	No

to kill most bacteria, viruses and fungi very effectively, but their action on *Mycobacterium tuberculosis* has yet to be proven. They are also user friendly. These compounds have been extensively used in the veterinary profession and hold a great deal of promise for surface disinfection: they are not recommended for immersion as they blacken instruments. As yet they have no EPA rating.

Use of disinfectants

Decontamination of surfaces

There is considerable debate about the risk of cross infection from contaminated surfaces. Unless there is gross contamination, then the risk is probably small but still has to be taken into consideration.[4] In the office, therefore, it is important to define the contaminated areas and clean areas. This concept of defining areas is called 'zoning'. If the areas are defined, then the surfaces that need to be disinfected are limited and this saves office time. Defining zoned areas needs discipline from both the DA and dentist, to ensure that no overlap with clean areas occurs. The choice of clean and dirty zones is at the discretion of the dentist and DA and will depend on the office equipment. Some of the usual dirty zone areas are listed in *Table 5.5*. One area that is often overlooked is the head rest which, by virtue of its proximity to the mouth, becomes heavily contaminated. This area needs disinfecting. Some practices cover the head-rest area with polythene which is discarded after every patient.

Table 5.5   Usual dirty zone areas: some examples

Dirty	*Clean*
Bracket table	All other areas
Dentist's equipment	
Switches and control	
Head rest	
Light handle and switches	
Any cabinetry surfaces	
DA's equipment switches	

A good method of disinfecting surfaces is to spray the disinfectant on to the area, wipe it off and then spray it on again followed by a wipe. This achieves cleaning, dilution and then secondary disinfection.

Spillages

Gross spillages of blood, vomit or other *fomites* can present a problem in the surgery. It is important that a careful sequence of procedures is followed to ensure that no risk of cross infection occurs. The DA first puts on thick protective gloves and then covers the area with a disinfectant powder. Undiluted granules (for example gluteraldehyde) are useful for the purpose. The area is then left for at least 10 minutes before being cleaned with paper towels. After the first covering, as much particulate and liquid matter as possible is removed and placed into a bag for disposal. The process is repeated at least three times before the area is disinfected with a surface disinfectant. If the area cannot be isolated, then the same procedures are followed without any time between powder application and removal. In these circumstances, at least four or five applications are necessary to soak up the liquid part of the spillage. The applications are repeated with care until all visible material is removed. Surface disinfection is the final stage of the process.

Non-surgical instruments

Non-surgical instruments are best soaked in an EPA-recommended disinfectant for one hour and then thoroughly cleaned of all detritus. The instruments are then sprayed with a suitable surface disinfectant.

Dental-unit water supplies (DUWS)

Dental-unit water supplies become heavily contaminated from two sources. The first source is the water supply itself, particularly if it is derived from the mains. The second source is the retraction of material into the tubing of the DUWS when instruments such as the air and water syringe and the air turbine are deactivated. Many of the micro-organisms can be pathogenic in compromised patients.[5]

Once into the DUWS, the micro-organisms are difficult to remove as they form a biofilm on the tube linings. Running the water supply for five minutes has been advocated, but this only clears the contamination in the liquid phase of the DUWS. On deactivation, the DUWS are again contaminated by oral micro-organisms. Dental units with non-retraction valves are now being manufactured but these will only be useful if the water supply is clean. Clearly the ideal situation is to provide the units with microbe-free water and to sterilize all handpieces and air and water syringes.

A number of disinfection systems have now been designed to introduce antimicrobials into the DUWS. These are effective but do not obviate the need for sterilization of handpieces and air and water syringes. The use of contaminated DUWS is probably not significant to the majority of patients, but is contraindicated in the immunocompromised.

Decontamination of grossly contaminated areas

One area of the surgery that also becomes grossly contaminated is the spittoon, associated drains and the water-aspiration system. By virtue of the fact that patients rinse out and void the material into these areas, disinfection must be frequent and effective. Non-foaming disinfectants must be used in these areas at least at the beginning and end of every clinical session. The preferred disinfectant is gluteraldehyde of a buffered type, of at least double strength. This disinfectant is then followed by at least the equivalent volume of water. Mobile aspiration systems incorporating a bottle should contain at least one-third of their volume of disinfectant prior to use. This ensures that all aspirated material is mixed with disinfectant in situ. Aspirator bottles should be emptied frequently and long before they are full if accidents or spillages are to be avoided. Disposal should be down a drain not a sink.

Disinfection prior to sterilization

There is some merit in putting instruments into disinfection prior to cleaning and sterilization (holding baths). The phenolics are recommended for this purpose. This often kills some micro-organisms and minimizes hand scrubbing. It can often prevent airborne spread of microbes. Care must be exercised in removing the instruments from the holding disinfectant and long-handled tweezers should be used.

Disposal of contaminated waste

Two types of contaminated waste are generated from dental practice: sharps and other materials. Sharps need containment in rigid containers which cannot be punctured. They are filled no more than two-thirds full so that accidental needlestick injuries are avoided when sharps are placed in the container. Sharps containers should be incinerated.

Most regulatory bodies in the USA and the UK now require that other materials generated during clinical procedures should be incinerated. These materials are put into stout bags clearly marked with 'contaminated material – to be incinerated'. Local arrangements have to be made for this incineration.

Decontamination of instruments prior to servicing

In the UK and certain parts of Europe, it is now mandatory to decontaminate instruments or equipment prior to their servicing. Decontamination of such instruments as turbines can be done by autoclaving. Other fixed pieces of equipment must be decontaminated with suitable EPA-recommended surface disinfectants. These procedures protect service engineers.

6

Auxiliary personnel and cross infection control

The auxiliary personnel in dentistry are important members of the cross infection control team. They must be fully trained in the techniques of cross infection control and understand why the procedures are being done. In an ideal world this would involve a full infection-control training programme prior to any office exposure. In some centres this is done, but it is the exception rather than the rule. Most new personnel are in fact trained by existing staff, either by observation or actually on the job. The end-result depends on the quality of the teacher and what steps are taken to remedy any resultant errors.

Problems can arise when infection-control measures are introduced to staff who have been employed for some time and who are inflexible and resistant to change. Here the resistance to change can be pronounced and difficult to manage. In this author's experience, failure to wear protective glasses and gloves is perhaps the most common manifestation of this problem. Great care and tact are necessary in this situation if the co-operation of a valuable and important worker is not to be alienated. It must be stressed that co-operation must be achieved if the practice is to be safe.

One of the simplest methods of avoiding problems is to ensure that the initial contract of employment contains some mention of cross infection control measures. The insertion of a clause to the effect that 'The employee shall use such cross infection control measures as directed by the employer' avoids any ambiguity and allows flexibility for future developments. This also avoids problems of a more costly nature when any dispute occurs over dismissal. Such claims for unfair dismissal have been tested in the courts in both the UK and the USA. In many of the cases, the litigation could have been shortened or aborted if a *written* contract containing some mention of cross infection control had been given to the employee.

Dental hygienist

With the exception of minor oral surgery, the duties of the hygienist offer a high potential risk of cross infection. This is as a direct consequence of the aerosols and splatter generated during scaling and polishing. The risk is increased in some countries where hygienists can work without direct supervision from a qualified dentist. In most Western countries, the work of a hygienist is still by direct prescription from a dentist. As for any other employee, the responsibility for cross infection control by the hygienist is directly attributable to the dentist. Clearly it is impossible for the dentist continually to supervise the work of the hygienist. It is therefore necessary to review periodically the cross infection control measures being undertaken.

Two particular areas of a dental hygienist's work are especially associated with risk of infection. The first is the practice of wiping calculus or other material from scalers with handheld napkins. This practice is best avoided as the risk of needlestick injury is high. The second is ultrasonic scaler tips which are often never sterilized. Ultrasonic scaler tips must be sterilized as they are usually grossly blood contaminated. With the majority of scaler tips, this will reduce their effective working life as they are deleteriously affected by heat. Certain scaler tips perform better than others and these differences are cost related.

Dental technician

The dental technician is potentially at risk from cross infection.[1] With care this risk can be reduced to practically nil.[2,3] This is done by ensuring a careful regimen for the transportation and treatment of all technical work that is to be sent to the laboratory. The expert advisory groups from a number of countries have made recommendations as to how this is to be achieved and detailed advice on the decontamination of impression materials, prostheses, orthodontic appliances, crowns, bridges and other appliances as well as guides to laboratory practice are now available.

Impression materials of various kinds have been evaluated for their stability when decontamination procedures are used. From *Table 6.1*, it can be seen that impression materials must be treated with specific disinfectants if their dimensional stability is not to be affected. Perhaps the most important part of the decontamination procedure is

Table 6.1   Impression materials: methods of decontamination

Impression material	*Method*	*Disinfectant*
Compound	Discard	
Agar	Wash in water and spray on disinfectant	All affect dimensional stability; spray with EPA-recommended disinfectant
Addition silicone	Wash in water and then immerse for 60 minutes	Immerse in 2 per cent (w/v) gluteraldehyde or hypochlorite (10 000 ppm chlorine)
Condensation silicone	Wash in water and then immerse for 60 minutes	Immerse in 2 per cent (w/v) gluteraldehyde or hypochlorite (10 000 ppm chlorine)
Polysulphur	Wash in water and then immerse for 60 minutes	Immerse in 2 per cent (w/v) gluteraldehyde or hypochlorite (10 000 ppm chlorine)
Polyether	Wash in water and spray	Spray with an EPA-recommended disinfectant
Zinc oxide/eugenol	Wash in water and then immerse for 60 minutes	Immerse in 2 per cent (w/v) gluteraldehyde

to wash the impression carefully under running water until all traces of blood, saliva or other organic material have been removed. The most difficult of all the impression materials to decontaminate are alginate and other irreversible hydrocolloids. At present there is no solution, although impregnation with disinfectants such as didecyldimethyl ammonium chloride has been tried but its effects are not proven. Prostheses, orthodontic appliances, crowns and bridges should all be carefully washed before being taken into the laboratory for technical work. Ultrasonic cleaning for two minutes is a useful first step. Dentures and orthodontic appliances can be immersed in sodium hypochlorite for four minutes. A designated dirty area should be reserved for receipt of this material. Crown and bridge material is best adjusted at the chair side. If reglazing is necessary, then the oven temperature (circa 1000°C) will kill all micro-organisms.

Care should be taken in laboratories to clean all surfaces with a suitable EPA-approved disinfectant. Polishing mops should be regularly cleaned and burs and grinding wheels should be sterilized at least every week. It is important to change pumice regularly and to wear masks and eye protection when polishing. Finished materials can be washed carefully. In the USA, gas sterilization with ethylene oxide for 45 minutes is useful. Gas sterilizers are expensive to buy and need careful maintenance. The appliance is stored dry in a sealed polythene bag, and should be washed carefully at the chair side prior to fitting.

The safety of the laboratory depends on good laboratory practice. All material brought into it should be regarded as potentially infective and clean and dirty areas should always be respected. Needless to say, no eating, drinking or smoking should be allowed in any laboratory and hand washing should be done at least before and after work.

Office cleaner

In every office, there should be a definite policy as to who cleans and disinfects each area. It is preferable for the dental units, light, chair, working surfaces and sinks to be cleaned by the DA. All other surfaces, especially the floors, can be cleaned by the cleaner. Floors do become heavily contaminated as material under the influence of gravity does fall. Damp mops impregnated with a detergent are suitable for this job. The addition of a compatible disinfectant is useful. Cleaning of floors and other parts of the office is best done after the working session, not first thing in the morning. The choice of this time means that aerosols and other airborne particles are allowed to settle. All clean zones which are used for office materials should be covered with paper or other material.

Receptionist

The member of staff who would be thought least at risk from cross infection is the receptionist. Close contact with the patients is minimal and a safe working distance can be maintained. One method whereby infection can be transmitted is on record cards. Herpes simplex type I virus has been transmitted on record cards and it is therefore important that they are kept in non-contaminated zones of the office and not touched until surgery is finished and hands have been disinfected.

Infection control in specialized practice

In the preceding chapters, cross infection control measures have been discussed which relate to routine general dental practice. In this chapter, the specialized areas of oral surgery, periodontology, orthodontics and the treatment of the immunocompromised will be discussed.

Oral surgery

Oral surgery requires cross infection control measures in addition to those practised for other forms of general dentistry. The reason for this is that many of the procedures carried out are elective and therefore infection is an unnecessary complication. Practitioners undertaking oral surgery need to be sure that their auxiliary personnel are trained to a high standard in oral surgery procedures. Poor technique by either the DA or the operator can result in infection. It has been stated that most of the postoperative infections that occur in any branch of surgery are caused at the time of operation. Some of these can result from poor technique.

It is perhaps axiomatic that everything used in oral surgery must be sterile and that contamination must be reduced to the minimum. Gloves should be sterile and discarded after use or if punctured. Ideally gowns and masks should be worn. Many oral surgeons also wear surgery-type hats to cover their hair, although the evidence that this prevents cross infection in oral surgery is lacking.

It is difficult to sterilize the site of operation during oral surgery, but the use of pre-operative chlorhexidine 0.2 per cent (w/v) is effective. This antiseptic can be used either to swab the operation area before incision or as an irrigant around the gingival crevice. In these sites it can help to reduce bacterial contamination or dry sockets respectively.[1,2] The use of chlorhexidine as an irrigant before extraction also reduces bacteraemias in patients susceptible to infective endocarditis.[3] Chlorhexidine is also thought to decrease the pathogenicity of some Gram-negative bacteria.

The irrigant and coolant solutions used in oral surgery must not only be sterile but also uncontaminated with proteinaceous matter. Contaminants such as microbial cell walls can be found in many drinking waters and these can act in an endotoxin-like fashion. In these circumstances, they could cause pain, delayed healing or wound dehiscence. It is therefore important to use distilled water if it is to be sterilized in the practice.

All gowns and coverings must be sterile. Paper coverings are convenient as they can be discarded after use. Surgical cloths can be used but any traces of blood must be washed from them prior to sterilization. This can be achieved by first washing the articles in a domestic washing machine, preferably at a temperature above 60°C, and then sterilizing them in an autoclave with a drying cycle. Many oral surgeons find such procedures cumbersome and prefer to use disposable materials such as paper products.

Many of the instruments used in oral surgery are of necessity sharp. They will also be blood-contaminated. A useful measure prior to sterilization is to immerse them in fresh 2 per cent (w/v) gluteraldehyde for one hour prior to two minutes of ultrasonic cleaning. This procedure kills many micro-organisms and reduces the risks from needlestick injuries. Any such injuries should be treated immediately as described on pages 20–1.

Periodontology

Many of the problems of cross infection control in periodontology are common to those of oral surgery. There is, however, some evidence that micro-organisms can be transferred from one pocket to another, since the flora is site-specific. However, there is no evidence that this causes a type of endogenous cross infection; there is therefore no need to change instruments for each site.

Orthodontics

The specialist practice of orthodontics has undergone a minor revolution in the last decade. There has been an increase in the number of fixed appliances used and a concomitant decrease in the use of removable appliances. The application of fixed appliances and their removal is often accompanied by contamination with saliva and blood, particularly in experienced hands! This change in practice has also been accompanied by an increase in the age range of patients treated. Adult orthodontic treatment, formerly a rarity, is now relatively commonplace. Some of the adult patients may be 'risk' groups. It necessarily follows that cross infection control measures in orthodontics must be as good as for any other branch of dentistry.

There are, however, problems with such a simple approach to cross infection control in orthodontics. The first problem is the orthodontists themselves who do not perceive cross infection control as a problem. In general, there is at present low compliance with cross infection control procedures amongst orthodontists.

Another major problem is that, if instruments are to be sterilized, then the capital outlay required to provide sufficient quantities is large. Such capital outlays are unavoidable if sterile instruments are to be provided for each patient. The ideal situation is to provide a sterile set of instruments, designed for each procedure, for each patient. The sterilization procedures for these instruments are exactly comparable to those used for other instruments in terms of presterilization cleaning, sterilization and aseptic storage (Chapter 4).

Hot-air sterilization is not recommended for orthodontic instruments as it tempers them and causes them to fracture. The ideal sterilization procedure is with hot vapours in the chemiclave. This does not rust or corrode the instruments and causes the minimum deleterious effects on cutting edges and moving joints. Immersion in disinfectants is not recommended for orthodontic instruments as it causes corrosion and joint stiffness of instruments such as pliers. Autoclaving is useful for orthodontic instruments but it can cause corrosion and dullness. This can be avoided by washing the instruments in distilled water, lubricating them and then dipping them in a reducing agent such as 2 per cent (w/v) sodium nitrite prior to autoclaving.

Cross infection control in orthodontics does require teamwork. To prevent contamination of elastics, ligatures and archwires, a simple aseptic transfer from containers must be used by the DA. With practice, this can be achieved. A strict zone system must be used with surface disinfection on the completion of each patient.

Patients who are to have removable appliances fitted or adjusted should also have sterile instruments used on them. A kit for the adjustment of removable appliances should be devised and sterilized. Adjustments of acrylic appliances should be done in the same way as for dentures.

It has been stated above, but bears repetition, that cross infection control is as important in orthodontics as in any other branch of dentistry. At present, some of the instruments that are used are not technologically ideal for such procedures as sterilization. It is to be hoped that future developments in the manufacture of these instruments will solve these problems.

Immunocompromised patients

An immunocompromised patient has impaired body defences and is therefore susceptible to infection. Thus even contamination with micro-organisms whose numbers are below the minimum infective dose can result in serious and often life-threatening infection. The necessity for good infection control when treating these patients cannot be overstressed.

Table 7.1 shows a list of patients who may be immunocompromised. This list is not exhaustive and often transient immunosuppression

Table 7.1   Immunocompromised patients

Cause	Examples
Physiological	Neonates
	Old age
Drug-induced	Cytotoxic agents
	Antimetabolic agents
Autoimmune disease	Diabetes mellitus
	Rheumatoid arthritis
Malignant disease	Leukaemia
	Hodgkin's disease
Radiotherapy	

PRACTICAL POINTS
—additional cross infection control for immunocompromised patients

- **Use all the cross infection control procedures for a non-compromised patient**
- **Use sterile distilled water for all cooling and irrigation purposes**
- **Avoid minor oral surgery if possible**
- **If minor oral surgery is necessary use pre-operative disinfection and prophylactic antimicrobial agents**
- **Refer for a specialist opinion if necessary**
- **Liaise with the patient's physician in *all* cases**

may follow any debilitating illness or is a consequence of old age. It will be noted from *Table 7.1* that the potential list of the immunocompromised is large and growing, particularly with the AIDS pandemic and the administration of anti-rejection drugs for transplantation. What is important to note is that the majority of immunocompromised patients can live life outside hospitals, provided that they take reasonable precautions not to become infected.

Immunocompromised patients can become infected by dental procedures. Precautions taken for any non-compromised patient are suitable for these susceptible individuals, but other measures must be added. One of the most important of these is to use sterile distilled water for all cooling and irrigant purposes. Dental-unit water supplies may contain Gram-negative micro-organisms that may contaminate the patient and lead to infection.

HIV-antibody-positive, AIDS-related-complex and AIDS patients

The pandemic of HIV transmission in the world has led to a new set of cross infection control problems for dentistry. Many dentists have simply reacted by stating that they would refuse to treat an HIV-antibody-positive patient. Such attitudes are safe only as long as the patient volunteers the information that he or she is infected. The cross infection control measures described in this book are designed to be safe for any patient, including those infected with HIV or the hepatitis viruses. In the opinion of most expert groups, HIV-antibody-positive patients can be treated by general dental practitioners. The aim of treatment is to bring their oral health and hygiene to a satisfactory state and to maintain it. If the patient develops AIDS or ARC then more specialist treatment may be required and referral should be considered.

Office routine

In the preceding chapter, the principles and details of cross infection control have been discussed. This chapter is designed to give a checklist of the routines that are used to ensure safe, reproducible cross infection control for the general practitioner. The sections are split into the duties of the DA and the dentist.

At the start of the day

DA

- Don heavy-duty gloves, spectacles, protective apron and mask
- Disinfect clean and dirty areas with surface disinfectant
- Disinfect spittoon
- Wash heavy-duty gloves and take them off
- Consult clinical notes for the first patient
- Full hand wash
- Don operating gloves, spectacles and mask
- Lay out instruments
- Wash hands, then open instrument trays

Dentist

- Full hand wash
- Consult notes
- Don gloves, spectacles and mask
- Wash gloves
- Operate on patient

On the completion of treatment

Dentist

- Wash or discard gloves
- Write up case notes

DA

- Remove instruments
- Sharps to sharps box
- Clinical soiled waste to receiver box
- Don heavy-duty gloves
- Disinfect all contaminated areas
- Wash and remove heavy-duty gloves
- Don operating gloves

Repeat procedures as for the start of the day.

At the end of the day

DA

- Remove operating gloves, put on heavy-duty gloves
- Remove clinical waste and seal, send for incineration
- Disinfect all surfaces
- Disinfect aspiratal spittoon
- Remove heavy-duty gloves after washing

References

Introduction

1 *Health and Safety at Work Act* (HM Stationery Office, United Kingdom: London 1988).

2 The control of cross infection in dentistry, *Br Dent J* (1988) **165**:353–4.

3 American Dental Association Council on Dental Therapeutics and Council on Prosthetic Services and Dental Laboratory Relations, Guidelines for Infection Control in the Dental Office and the Commercial Dental Laboratory, *J Am Dent Assoc* (1985) **110**:969–72.

4 Centers for Disease Control, Recommended infection-control practices for dentistry, *Morbidity, Mortality, Weekly Report (MMWR)* (1986) **35**:237–42.

Chapter 1

1 Levin ML, Maddrey WC, Wands JR, Hepatitis B transmission by dentists, *JAMA* (1974) **228**:1139–40.

2 Grady GF, Hepatitis B from medical professionals how rare? How preventable? *N Engl J Med* (1977) **296**:995–6.

3 Rimland D, Parkin WE, Miller GB et al, Hepatitis B outbreak traced to an oral surgeon, *N Engl J Med* (1977) **296**:950–3.

4 Williams SV, Pattison CP, Berquist KR, Dental infection with hepatitis B, *JAMA* (1975) **232**:1231–3.

5 Kew MC, Possible transmission of serum hepatitis via the conjunctiva, *Infect Immun* (1973) **7**:823–4.

6 Pattison CP, Maynard JE, Endemic hepatitis in a clinical laboratory, *JAMA* (1974) **230**:854–7.

7   Alter HJ, Purcell RH, Gerin JL, Transmission to chimpanzees by hepatitis B surface antigen positive saliva and serum, *Infect Immun* (1977) **16**:928–33.

8   Bancroft WH, Smithban, Scott RM, Transmission of hepatitis B virus to gibbons by exposure to human saliva containing hepatitis B surface antigen, *J Infect Dis* (1977) **135**:70–85.

9   Fevero MS, Hepatitis B on environmental surfaces, *Lancet* (1973) **ii**:1455.

10 Manzella JP, McConville JH, Valent N et al, An outbreak of herpes simplex type I gingivostomatitis in a dental hygiene practice, *JAMA* (1984) **252**:2019–22.

11 Linnemann CC, Buchman TG, Light IJ et al, Transmission of herpes simplex virus type I in a nursery for the newborn: identification of viral isolates by DNA 'fingerprinting', *Lancet* (1978) **i**:964–6.

12 Mintz GA, Klocko K, Cutarelli P et al, Survival of herpes simplex on dental handpieces, *J Oral Med* (1985) **40**:158–9.

13 US Department of Health and Human Services, Public Health Service, *Preventing the Transmission of Hepatitis B, AIDS and Herpes in Dentistry* (CDC: Georgia 1989).

14 Porter SR, Scully C, Cawson RA, AIDS: update and guidelines for dental practice, *Dent Update* (1987) **14**:9–17.

15 Autio KL, Rosen S, Reynolds NJ et al, Studies on cross contamination in the dental clinic, *J Am Dent Assoc* (1980) **100**:358–61.

16 Martin MV, The significance of the bacterial contamination of dental unit water systems, *Br Dent J* (1987) **162**:459–62.

17 Martin MV, Hardy P, Multiply resistant *Staphylococcus aureus* in dental patients, *Br Dent J* (1990) in press.

18 Smith RA, Hitchcock CA, Evans EGV et al, The identification of *Candida albicans* strains by restriction fragment length polymorphism analysis of DNA, *J Med Vet Mycol* (1989) **27**:431–4.

19 Mitchell R, Russell J, The elimination of cross infection in dental practice – a five year follow up, *Br Dent J* (1989) **166**:209–11.

20 Glenwright HD, Shovelton DS, The prevention of cross infection: progress in the West Midlands, *Br Dent J* (1989) **166**:125–7.

Chapter 3

1   Council on Dental Materials, Instruments and Equipment, Infection control for the dental office and dental laboratory, *J Am Dent Assoc* (1988) **116**:241–8.

2 Editorial, The control of cross infection in dentistry, *Br Dent J* (1988) **165**:353–4.

3 Field EA, King C, Dermatological problems associated with the routine wearing of gloves by dentists, *Br Dent J* (1990) in press.

4 Allen AL, Organ RJ, Occult blood accumulation under the fingernails; a mechanism for the spread of blood borne infection, *J Am Dent Assoc* (1982) **105**:455–9.

5 Ayliffe GA, Babb JR, Quoradishi AH, A test for hygienic hand disinfection, *J Clin Pathol* (1978) **31**:923–8.

6 Field EA, Martin MV, Handwashing: soap or disinfectant? *Br Dent J* (1980) **160**:278–80.

7 Holloway PM, Bucknall RA, Denton GW, The effects of sublethal contents of chlorhexidine on bacterial pathogenicity, *J Hosp Infect* 8:39–42.

8 Field EA, Martin MV, Disinfection of dental surgeons' hands with detergent preparations of triclosan and chlorhexidine, *J Dent* (1986) **14**:7–10.

9 Rotter ML, Koller W, Wewalka G et al, Evaluation of procedures for hygienic hand-disinfection controlled parallel experiments on the Vienna test model, *J Hyg (Camb)* (1986) **96**:27–37.

10 Martin MV, Dunn HM, Field EA et al, A physical and microbiological evaluation of the reuse of non-sterile gloves, *Br Dent J* (1988) **165**:321–4.

11 Kew MC, Possible transmission of serum hepatitis via the conjunctiva, *Infect Immun* (1973) **7**:823–4.

12 Micik RE, Miller RL, Leong AC, Studies in dental aerobiology III: Efficacy of surgical masks in protecting dental personnel from airborne bacterial particles, *J Dent Res* (1971) **50**:626–30.

13 Craig DC, Quayle AA, The efficacy of face masks, *Br Dent J* (1985) **158**:87–90.

14 Orr NWM, Is a mask necessary in the operating theatre? *Ann R Coll Surg Engl* (1981) **63**:390–1.

15 Siegel LJ, Smith KE, Infection control barrier techniques used by physicians during routine examinations: parental attitudes, *Clin Pediatr* (1989) **28**:231–4.

16 Rustrage KJ, Rothwell PS, Brook IM, Evaluation of a dedicated dental procedure glove for clinical dentistry, *Br Dent J* (1987) **163**:193–5.

17 Mitchell R, Cumming CG, Maclennan WD et al, The use of operating gloves in dental practice, *Br Dent J* (1983) **154**:272–4.

Chapter 4

1   Martin MV, The sterilization of instruments in dental practice. In: Derrick D, ed. *The dental annual* (Butterworths: Kent 1988) 188–95.

2   Johnson G, Perry F, Pellan G, Effect of four anticorrosive drips on the cutting efficiency of dental carbide burs, *J Am Dent Assoc* (1978) **97**:628–32.

3   Hurst V, Reducing the risk of transmitting viral hepatitis via dental instruments, *J Dent Res* (1972) **52**:150.

4   Wilson G, Bacterial resistance, disinfection and sterilization. In: Wilson G, Miles A, Parker MT, eds. *Topley and Wilson's Principles of Bacteriology, Virology and Immunity* 7th edn, Vol 1 (Edward Arnold: London 1983).

5   Martin MV, Bartzokas CA, The boiling of instruments in dental practice: a monomer for sterilization, *Br Dent J* (1985) **159**:18–20.

6   Shorelton DS, Glenwright HD, Bradnock G, Precautions taken by a group of dentists in West Midlands against cross infection, *Br Dent J* (1987) **163**:383–6.

7   Woods PR, Martin MV, A study of the use of autoclave bags in non-vacuum autoclaves, *J Dent* (1989) **17**:148–9.

8   Field EA, Field JK, Martin MV, Time Steam Temperature (TST) control indicators to measure essential sterilization criteria for autoclaves in general dental practice and the community dental services, *Brit Dent J* (1988) **164**:183–6.

Chapter 5

1   Block SS, *Sterilization, Disinfection and Preservation*, 3rd edn (Lea and Febiger: Philadelphia 1983).

2   Wilson G, Bacterial resistance disinfection and sterilization. In: Wilson G, Miles A, Parker MT, eds. *Topley and Wilson's Principles of Bacteriology, Virology and Immunity*, 7th edn, Vol 1 (Edward Arnold: London 1983) 7–96.

3   US Environmental Protection Agency, Tuberculocidal test method, *Data Call in Notices for Tuberculicidal Effectiveness* (Washington DC: US Environmental Protection Agency, Disinfectants Branch, Registration Division 1988) 1–6.

4   Christensen RP, Robinson RA, Robinson DF et al, Antimicrobial activity of environmental surface disinfectants in the absence and presence of bioburden, *J Am Dent Assoc* (1989) **119**:493–505.

5 Martin MV, The significance of the bacterial contamination of dental unit waste supplies, *Br Dent J* (1987) **162**:459–62.

Chapter 6

1 Sabitini BM, Don't let it happen to you, *NADLJ* (1982) **29**:19–23.

2 Centers for Disease Control, Recommendations, infection control practices for dentistry, *MMWR* (1986) **34**:313–35.

3 Council on Dental Materials, Infection control recommendations for the dental office and dental laboratory, *J Am Dent Assoc* (1988) **116**:241–8.

Chapter 7

1 Field EA, Nind DA, Varga E et al, The effects of irrigation on the incidence of dry socket: a pilot study, *Br J Oral Max Surg* (1988) **26**: 390–5.

2 Martin MV, Nind D, A study of chlorhexidine gluconate for preoperative disinfection of apicetomy sites, *Br Dent J* (1987) **162**:459–62.

3 MacFarlane TW, Ferguson MM, Mulgrew CJ, Postextraction bacteraemia role of antiseptics and antibiotics, *Br Dent J* (1984) **156**:179–81.

Index